ANTICANCER
The Preventive Power of Food

ANTICANCER
The Preventive Power of Food

A Nutrition Guide to Reduce Cancer Risk

Christina Economidou Pieridou

ISBN: 978-9963-2353-0-8

Christina Economidou Pieridou
My Nutrilosophy
christina@mynutrilosophy.com
5 Korrinis street, 4043, Limassol, Cyprus

Edited by Sandra J. Judd

Disclaimer

The information contained in this book is not intended nor implied to be a substitute for professional medical advice, it is provided for educational purposes only. Readers should always seek the advice of a professional physician or other qualified healthcare provider before starting any new treatment or discontinuing an existing treatment. Readers need also to talk with their healthcare provider about any questions they may have regarding a medical condition. Nothing contained in these topics is intended to be used for medical diagnosis, cure or treatment and/or mitigation or prevention of any type of disease or medical condition.

The information and materials provided in this book are based upon the professional experience and extensive academic research carried out by the author and are only meant to supplement the information that readers obtain from their qualified healthcare providers.

Readers should further recognize that the information and materials presented in this book will be beneficial to the majority of people, however, as any individual has his own personal needs, arising from their family history, current and past health status and many other factors, the same information may not be applicable to any reader's particular case.

Readers should promptly consult their physician or other healthcare provider and never disregard medical or professional advice, or delay seeking it, because of something they read in this book, as well as, they must never rely on information in the same book in place of seeking professional medical advice, but they should also ask their physician or other healthcare provider to assist them in interpreting any information in this book or in the linked websites, or in applying the information to their individual case.

Readers assume full responsibility for how they choose to use this information and materials. Besides, the author is not liable or responsible for any advice, course of treatment, diagnosis or any other information, services or product readers obtain through this book.

My Nutrilosophy

My Nutrilosophy was created in 2014 by three registered dietitians, Tina Christoudias, Vanessa Xenopoulou and Christina Economidou. With twenty years of experience in the field of nutrition, they founded **My Nutrilosophy** out of their passion to exceed the boundaries of their profession and to seek a more holistic nutritional approach to health.

The new nutrition philosophy they are advocating is based on cutting edge scientific evidence and aims to promote the healing power of real food, to help the body heal from within and to integrate natural and traditional therapies with modern science.

The mission of My Nutrilosophy is to provide science-based nutrition information that will help people improve their health.

You can access all this information by visiting ~~www.mynutrilosophy.com.~~ www.nutritioncanheal.com In the website you will find:

- the latest research on diet and cancer,
- recipes that help in the prevention of cancer,
- nutrition packages,
- great resources on many other health topics.

Join My Nutrilosophy community and start transforming your health.

About the Author

Christina Economidou Pieridou is a clinical dietitian and nutritionist. She has a B.Sc. from King's College London in Nutrition and Dietetics, and did her registration work for clinical dietetics in two big central London hospitals. She also holds an M.Sc. in Nutritional Medicine from the University of Surrey which is one of the leading courses in nutrition science globally.

She practices as a clinical dietitian in Cyprus since 2000.

Her journey as a dietitian and nutritional therapist took a different turn when My Nutrilosophy was created in 2014. Teaming up with her friends and colleagues Tina and Vanessa helped her realize it was the right time to open up to more natural, holistic and integrative approaches in nutritional therapy.

Through her practice she has helped thousands of people and small children to support their health with good nutrition and to cope with serious health problems.

"Anticancer – The Preventive Power of Food" is Christina's second book. In 2012 she wrote her first book "How to become Your Own Dietitian". The book was published by an established Greek publishing company and sold thousands of copies.

Christina has always been very passionate about spreading the message of good nutrition. She has participated in large government funded health promotion programs in her community. Between the years 2006 and 2016 she ran her own website on nutrition and health issues. Throughout her career she gave countless lectures, seminars, workshops and interviews on a great number of nutrition topics and she is especially passionate about teaching healthy eating habits to children.

CONTENTS

PART A
Introduction to Cancer

PART B
Weight–Cancer Link

PART E
Avoid the Foods that Promote Cancer

PART F
Toxin Removal and Physical Activity

ACKNOWLEDGMENTS

I would like to thank my two My Nutrilosophy colleagues, friends and partners, Tina and Vanessa for creating such a great energy in our team and for sharing the same passion for continuous learning and the need to spread our findings to the world through My Nutrilosophy. I would also like to thank my friend Charis Michael for believing in our team's philosophy from the first instant and for her continuous support.

Additionally, I would like to thank my family for their constant support while I was writing this book. They helped me find the time to concentrate on my research and writing. I also owe a special thanks to my close friends who are a great inspiration for natural living.

Most importantly, I want to express my gratitude to the hundreds of visionaries, scientists, and researchers who have contributed to the scientific knowledge that is available today in the field of nutrition and cancer. With my book I try to bring their work closer to the world and to help in creating a cancer-free world.

THE FAMILY STORY THAT BROUGHT
ME CLOSE TO CANCER

A few years ago we found out that my cousin had been diagnosed with cancer. A bright scientist who was then doing her post-doc research in pharmacology, she was thirty-four at the time.

She immediately flew home to have her treatments done close to her family. I remember our discussions with her mother about what she could eat—that is, what would be the best diet for her while she was doing her chemotherapy sessions.

The six months that followed will always hold a very special place in my heart. In my weekly visits to Daina I rediscovered her amazing character, her tranquility and calmness, and her huge smiles and endless courage. Being there for her was the only thing that made sense and that made me feel good during those six months.

MY QUEST FOR A BETTER UNDERSTANDING
OF THE ROLE OF NUTRITION ON CANCER

I remember speaking with Daina's sister about natural dietary treatments that other cancer patients were following. These natural approaches suggested avoiding sugar, eating mostly organic whole foods, and taking specific nutritional supplements. Their aim was to protect the parts of the body that were still healthy and to enhance the body's natural defense mechanisms in order to help it fight the disease.

As a clinical dietitian who was trained and worked in two big central London hospitals in the late nineties, I had the opportunity to work in the oncology departments. There, I was trained to follow the hospital's protocols, which involved supporting patients' cancer treatments nutritionally. I was taught to prescribe high-sugar dietary supplements to help maintain weight and prevent weight loss. Having thus been taught otherwise in my training and first dietetic job, hearing at the time of Daina's illness that sugar actually feeds cancer came as a big surprise to me.

After I left London, my career focused on promoting healthy nutrition habits, on both a personal and a community level. I worked on promoting long-term health and disease prevention. I knew that Western diets, loaded with excess sugar, were related to the world's obesity and cancer epidemics. Yet when it came to cancer and nutrition, I began to realize that there was a lot of new scientific knowledge that was waiting for me to explore.

My journey as a dietitian and nutritional therapist took a different turn when our team, My Nutrilosphy, was created. As a team of three clinical dietitians with the best academic backgrounds and with fifteen-plus years of practice, we all felt it was the right time to open up to more natural and integrative approaches. From our first meeting we all realized that we shared the same passion for exploring new therapeutic approaches and integrating them in our dietetic practice.

Once we got together, the three of us embarked on a mission of continuous study. Our aim was to combine our clinical dietetic knowledge with the wisdom of older approaches like herbal medicine and with more natural approaches. Along the way we discovered and shared exciting findings of new cutting-edge scientific studies that provide evidence for the therapeutic value of specific herbs, foods, and of modern dietary approaches.

Our team's new nutrition philosophy, *nutrilosophy*, describes our passion for finding quality scientific data on natural approaches that will help people adopt a new lifestyle and new eating habits that will help minimize risks to their health. In other words, we want to give people the tools to offer their body the optimum nutrition, in order to improve long-term health and, when needed, help the body repair itself.

Most of the new information I came across on this fascinating educational journey was related to cancer. My strong emotions related to the recent loss of a loved and very young family member to cancer focused my interest and guided me toward learning more about this disease.

My initial search on the topic was an eye-opener. I then began to study the work of doctors and researchers in centers throughout the world that were offering complementary or holistic approaches to cancer patients. They all incorporated nutrition in their protocols in order to help the body develop a strong immune system that would help in the healing process.

Shortly after I started my focused research on cancer, I was asked to give a talk on nutrition and cancer prevention by a good friend from a local association for cancer. The people who attended the talk were very enthusiastic about the information they were given. They were inspired by the fact that improving their diets could significantly reduce the risk of getting cancer. They were also happy to learn that good nutrition could increase the possibility of treating cancer successfully, as they learned about everyday foods that have strong anti-cancer properties.

This experience increased my excitement about being able to share my new findings and deepened my search on the link between diet and cancer. The findings of this search are presented in this book with the hope that I may reach and help as many people as possible.

HOW THIS BOOK CAN HELP

This book is the result of a thorough review of a great number of scientific studies that link cancer with dietary choices. In this book I will share with you the latest research on how the food we eat can either promote or block the initiation and progression of cancer.

In the last few decades, scientists have discovered numerous powerful anticancer compounds that are found naturally in many common foods. These foods and their anticancer compounds will be thoroughly analyzed in this book, which will also teach you ways to use diet to support your immune system in order to boost its potential to defend the body against cancer.

The book also presents a long list of the nutritional factors that promote the development of cancer. These include carcinogenic substances that are created by cooking at high temperatures, pollutants in fish, and bad fats. These carcinogenic substances are responsible for the development of cancer, and we should aim to reduce our exposure to them as much as possible.

Furthermore, this book presents the results of research on how particular foods can enhance the effectiveness and reduce the side effects of common cancer therapies and how these foods can block the spread of tumors and prevent metastasis.

I deeply hope that this book will help you change the way you choose your food and the way you think about your health and about cancer.

HOW YOU CAN USE THIS BOOK

The book presents the results of my in-depth research on the latest scientific evidence on the role of diet in cancer. Though I have presented the information in a specific order that I think will be useful, you may want to jump back and forth between the chapters that are most interesting or relevant to you.

As a general guide, I have organized the book as follows:

PART A:

In Chapter 1 I explain what cancer is, show how it develops and progresses, and describe the main characteristics of cancer cells. This knowledge will be useful in understanding the information presented in the following chapters.

Chapter 2 introduces the new science of epigenetics—a breakthrough scientific discovery that proves that a healthy diet and lifestyle can turn off cancer genes and turn on your cancer-fighting potential. You will read amazing research that proves that even in people with high genetic risk, optimum nutrition can be remarkably effective in preventing cancer.

PART B:

Chapter 3 analyzes the link between weight and cancer. You will soon understand how excess body fat, especially around the waist, causes several metabolic changes that promote cancer growth and development and how sugar intake, insulin resistance and inflammation are key players in increasing cancer risk.

Chapter 4 will help you appreciate the positive effects of controlling weight when a person is diagnosed with cancer and make you aware of the factors that might contribute to weight gain when receiving any of the common cancer treatments. This awareness together with the advice given in this chapter will help affected people optimize the results of their treatment.

PART C:

Chapter 5 shows how vitamin D has only just recently been recognized as playing a huge role in health promotion and cancer prevention, and Chapter 6 teaches you how to optimize your Vitamin D levels.

PART D:

Chapter 7 introduces the power of foods in the prevention of cancer.

In chapters 8 through 17 I present a long and detailed list of foods, herbs, oils, and enzymes that have been shown to have strong cancer-fighting properties. Each chapter closes with practical tips and advice for incorporating these protective agents in your daily diet.

Chapter 18 presents tips on cooking and food combinations for maximum cancer protection, and chapter 19 analyzes in more detail the newly discovered science of epigenetics. It describes the interaction between your diet and your genes and how this interaction influences the risk of cancer development.

PART E:

Chapters 20 through 27 present the foods, cooking methods, food additives, oils, and environmental toxins in the food chain that increase cancer risk. At the end of each chapter you will find a table with easy-to-follow and practical tips, for helping you minimize your exposure to these damaging foods.

PART F:

In Chapter 28 you will learn about detoxing. You will find lots of information and practical tips for enhancing toxin removal from your body so that you minimize the risk for potential damage from these toxins.

Lastly, in Chapter 29 I will discuss how exercise improves overall health and explain why it can be a strong weapon against cancer.

SELF ASSESSMENT OF NUTRITIONAL FACTORS FOR CANCER PREVENTION

By buying this book you are entering the worldwide community of My Nutrilosophy. As part of our commitment in helping you improve your health and helping in the prevention of cancer globally, we are inviting you to complete our online questionnaire. Our interactive questionnaire is intended as a self assessment tool that assesses the nutritional factors that are modifiable and that can impact your future health greatly by affecting cancer risk.

Our Anticancer Nutritional Self Assessment has been created in order to provide you with personalized tips and to help you concentrate on the specific actions you can take to improve your nutrition and optimize your diet's cancer preventive potential. To find the questionnaire follow the link below:

www.mynutrilosophy.com/anticancer/assessment

Simply visit the above link and answer the questions of the self assessment. After completing the assessment you will receive your personal 'Nutritional Factors Profile for Cancer Prevention' which will outline the recommended nutrition and lifestyle changes specific to you that will make the biggest impact on your cancer risk.

Once you obtain your personal 'Nutritional Factors Profile for Cancer Prevention' you can save or print it out for future reference.

PART A

Introduction
to Cancer

CHAPTER 1

What is Cancer

THERE ARE MORE THAN two hundred types of cancer. Cancer is the name given to a collection of related diseases that occur when cells become damaged and get out of control.

Cancer can start almost anywhere in the body, which is made up of trillions of cells. In all types of cancer, some of the body's cells begin to "rebel" and stop following the rules of healthy cells.

Healthy cells grow and divide to form new cells as the body needs them. Usually the body has just the right number of each type of cell. The body produces signals to control how much and how often cells divide. When cells grow old or become damaged, they die through a process called apoptosis and new cells take their place.

When cancer develops, however, this orderly process breaks down. Changes in the genetic code (DNA) of cells make them grow out of control. Cells with damaged DNA have the ability to escape apoptosis and survive. These cells then start dividing continuously and may eventually form a tumor.[1]

Many cancers form solid tumors, which are masses of tissue.[2] Cancers of the blood, such as leukemia, generally do not form solid tumors.

Cancerous tumors are malignant, which means they can spread into, or invade, other tissues. They break off and travel through the blood or the lymph system to distant places in the body, where they form new tumors far from the original tumor.

A significant factor that allows the survival of cancerous cells is their ability to form new blood vessels, a process known as angiogenesis. Angiogenesis allows them to have their own supply of oxygen and the nutrients necessary for their growth.

Characteristics of Cancer Cells:

1. Uncontrolled growth
2. Ignoring the signals to stop growth that are given by nearby healthy cells
3. Resistance to cell death (apoptosis)
4. Ability to form new blood vessels (angiogenesis), which allows a continuous supply of oxygen and nutrients to the tumor
5. Potential to divide and reproduce infinitely
6. Ability to invade the body's tissues and metastasize

CANCER TAKES YEARS TO FORM

Not all rebel cells lead to cancer. Out-of-order cell behavior happens regularly over one's lifespan, sometimes with no ill effects. Actually, cells that can develop into cancer are often present in our bodies; they're simply waiting for something to push them over the edge, to cause them to behave abnormally, to divide, to multiply, and to invade.

The development of cancer is gradual. The disease evolves over many years or even decades. This big time window in its development allows us an opportunity to intervene in order to keep potential tumors in a dormant state, preventing them from developing and maturing.

THE SAD TRUTH ABOUT CANCER STATISTICS AND PREDICTIONS

At a very early stage in my search on cancer I came across some heartbreaking cancer statistics.

Based on data presented by Cancer Research UK, in 2012 it was estimated that 14.1 million new cases of cancer occurred worldwide. Research carried out by the same organization predicts that the number of new cancer cases per year worldwide will rise to 23.6 million by 2030 (a 70 percent increase).[3]

Based on 2010–2012 data, approximately 40 percent of men and women will be diagnosed with cancer at some point in their lifetimes. This percentage was only 30 percent a few years ago, and is expected to rise to 50 percent within the next few decades.[4] In an analysis that was published in the British Journal of Cancer in 2015, it was concluded that in the next few years over half of people will face a cancer diagnosis at some point in their lives.

These statistics and predictions are alarming. They are numbers that cannot be ignored and that make us all realize the significance of prevention. Any information that helps you and your loved ones stay healthy, such as the information presented in this book, are precious because in most cases cancer is preventable.

CHAPTER 2

Is It All in the Genes or Do We Have the Chance to React?

CANCER IS INDEED A DISEASE that in the last few decades has become part of our lives. It affects so many people around us, within our own families, within our circle of friends, or among our coworkers. Some of you reading this book may even be struggling with cancer yourself.

So, what can we do? How do we react in this era when the incidence of cancer is increasing at an alarming rate? Do we continue living our lives believing that we have no power to affect our future health, or do we dare to become educated and take our health into our own hands?

There are many myths surrounding cancer. We're told, "It's in the genes," and, "it's inevitable if you have a family history." I've come across many people who don't believe lifestyle has any role in cancer development. In my discussions on the subject I often hear stories of people who smoked and lived up to one hundred years and of people who ate very healthily and exercised and still got cancer. Even oncologists very often tell their cancer patients that they can eat whatever they want and that diet does not affect their treatment outcomes and the progression of their disease, nor does it affect their family's chance of developing cancer too.

However, there is no scientific proof behind these claims. As you read this book you will discover for yourself that the chance of a person developing cancer is not just written in their genes but also written in their plates!

National and international institutions on cancer agree that only 5 to 10 percent of cancers are passed down from parents to children.[1,2]

The majority of cancers (90–95 percent) are caused by genetic changes that occur during our lifetimes and are triggered by our environment and lifestyle. Revolutionary researchers have discovered that our genes interact with our environment and with the foods we eat. Food is an important epigenetic modulator—it can change our DNA and how it is expressed, and it can basically turn the cancer genes on and off.[3]

It is a great relief to find out that a healthy lifestyle and a healthy diet can be remarkably effective in preventing many types of cancer. This diet-gene interaction can have a profound effect on one's risk of developing cancer and on preventing metastasis, the spread of cancer to other parts of the body.

The study described below is an inspiration to me, as it provides strong evidence that cancer is not just "written" in one's genes. It reinforces a very important message: that we all have a role in and responsibility for protecting our bodies against cancer with the choices we make.

OPTIMUM NUTRITION CAN BE SIGNIFICANTLY PROTECTIVE EVEN IN PEOPLE WITH HIGH GENETIC RISK

Dr. Parviz Ghadirian and his team at the University of Montreal studied a group of 738 women who had a harmful mutation in Breast Cancer Gene-1 (BRCA-1) and Breast Cancer Gene-2 (BRCA-2).[4] Mutations are changes in the structure and function of genes, which are inherited by our parents and are associated with increased risks of some types of cancer.

From the 738 women who participated in the study, 38 had been diagnosed with breast cancer. The rest were close relatives of the breast cancer patients who did a genetic screening for BRCA and in whom the BRCA gene mutation was identified. The study aimed to evaluate the possible interaction between genes and diet diversity in breast cancer risk.

The team examined the lifestyle and diet of those high-risk women through an interviewer-administered food frequency questionnaire. The questionnaire was developed by the National Cancer Institute of Canada and covered one year prior to the diagnosis of cancer.

The results of the study clearly suggest that the diversity of the fruits and vegetables in these women's diet had the power to change the risk status that was imprinted in their genes.

The women eating more fruit and vegetables had a lower risk of developing breast cancer. Those who ate more variety, up to twenty-seven different fruits and vegetables per week, had an amazing risk reduction of 73 percent compared with women carrying the same genes that had the least intake and poorest variety of fruit and vegetables.

What's even more inspiring and encouraging is that there is now a great volume of scientific research that shows that what we eat and how we choose to live our lives after being diagnosed with cancer can have a huge impact on the disease progression and on future health.

The interaction between diet and genes will be analyzed in more detail in chapter 20.

BALANCE BETWEEN CANCER-PROMOTING AND CANCER-PREVENTING FACTORS

More than half of the cancers occurring today are preventable by applying knowledge that is currently available to scientists. There are many modifiable risk factors related to the development of cancer. Primary among these are smoking, being overweight, lack of exercise, and an unhealthy diet.

When it comes to diet, a low intake of fruits and vegetables along with a high intake of refined Western foods, rich in sugar, salt, and bad fats, creates an internal environment that promotes cancer.

On the contrary, a carefully selected diet has the ability to boost the body's natural defenses against cancer. By strengthening the immune system, enhancing the body's ability to detoxify, reducing inflammation, and choosing a diet rich in natural anti-cancer molecules a person can fight cancer at its first stages of existence and increase the body's ability to stabilize tumors over very long periods of time.

So, in a person's lifetime, maintaining a balance between the cancer-promoting and the cancer-preventing factors will increase the body's ability to remain healthy and keep cancer away.

MOST CANCERS ARE PREVENTABLE

The World Health Organization (WHO) estimates that between 30 and 70 percent of cancers are preventable.[5,6] Data from other official sources, like the American Institute for Cancer Research (AICR), estimate that eating a healthy diet, being active, and maintaining a healthy weight can prevent as many as 35 to 40 percent of cancers.[7] The proportion of cancers that can be prevented is even higher for cancers of the gastrointestinal tract, reaching up to 70 percent. The AICR suggests that diet, weight, and physical activity are the three cornerstones of cancer prevention and advises people to do the following:

1. Choose mostly plant foods, limit red meat and avoid processed meat

2. Aim to be at a healthy weight throughout life

3. Be physically active every day in some way for thirty minutes or more.[8]

The AICR estimates that 33 percent of breast cancer cases can be prevented yearly in the United States through a healthy diet, regular physical activity, and being lean.[9] This is a hugely important estimation, as breast cancer is the most common cancer among women worldwide. This percentage is equivalent to 76,500 new breast cancer cases in US women per year.

Data from the same source estimate that as many as 50 percent of colorectal cancer cases can be prevented each year. Colorectal cancer is also very prevalent, being among the four most prevalent cancers in the world. In the United States alone, this estimation means that an extra 66,400 people could remain free of colorectal cancer per year simply by adopting a healthier lifestyle.

The AICR continues with estimations for other common cancers. A healthier lifestyle could prevent 59 percent of endometrial cancer cases, 47 percent of stomach cancer cases, 63 percent of mouth, pharyngeal, and laryngeal cancer cases, and 63 percent of cases of cancer of the esophagus.

I hope that you, like me, find the information you've read so far empowering. It is indeed great news that there are simple changes in one's lifestyle that can significantly reduce cancer risk. In the next chapters you will discover the most important lifestyle factors that are associated with a reduced cancer risk.

PART B

Weight–Cancer Link

CHAPTER 3

Reduce Cancer Risk by Maintaining a Healthy Weight

BEING OVERWEIGHT INCREASES THE RISK for some cancers. As noted in a recent position statement by the American Society of Clinical Oncology (ASCO), obesity is "quickly overtaking tobacco as the leading preventable cause of cancer".[1] This is particularly alarming, as the problem of obesity is taking on epidemic proportions and quickly spreading in developed and developing countries alike. Obesity affects people from all socioeconomic backgrounds and all age groups, even very young children.

Research analyzed by the World Health Organization shows that cancer mortality increases by 10 percent for each increase in category in the body mass index (BMI) (5 kg/m^2).[2] BMI is an indicator of weight category and can be calculated by dividing one's weight (in kg) by height (in meters) squared.

BMI = Weight (kg) / Height (m) ^{2}

WEIGHT CATEGORIES	BMI (kg/m²)
Underweight	<18.5
Healthy Weight	18.5-24.9
Overweight	25-29.9
Obese	30-34.9
Severely Obese	35-39.9
Morbidly Obese	>40

For men, changing weight category from healthy to overweight, from overweight to obese, and so on was associated with an increased risk of developing several cancers:

- esophageal cancer (50 percent higher risk)
- thyroid cancer (33 percent)
- colon cancer (25 percent)
- renal cancer (25 percent).

The corresponding data for women were:

- endometrial cancer (60 percent higher risk)
- gallbladder cancer (60 percent),
- esophageal cancer (50 percent)
- renal cancer (34 percent).

The list does not stop here, as other studies have also shown that excess body fat increases the risk for pancreatic cancer and postmenopausal breast cancer.[3]

In the United States, the American Institute for Cancer Research (AICR) has estimated that every year 110,000 cancer deaths are caused by obesity, making it the second leading cause of cancer deaths, behind smoking.[4]

THE WEIGHT- CANCER LINK

Weight affects cancer risk in many ways. In recent years researchers have begun to view cancer more as a metabolic disease than as a genetic one. Excess body fat, especially around the waist, causes several metabolic changes that promote cancer growth and development.

THE ROLES OF SUGAR AND INSULIN RESISTANCE

Sugar consumption per person has increased dramatically in the last few decades. Scientists see a clear link between high sugar consumption and the global rise in obesity and diabetes. In addition to being a major cause of obesity, there is increasing evidence that added dietary sugar increases the risk of developing type II diabetes and metabolic syndrome. As a result of these metabolic imbalances, the risk of cancer increases too.

Insulin resistance is the primary component of the metabolic syndrome. It occurs when excess fat deposited centrally in the body disables the action of insulin after meals, leading to blood sugar deregulation. Being overweight or obese gradually causes insulin resistance, resulting in high levels of both sugar and insulin in the blood for long periods of time. Insulin is a hormone that is responsible for promoting the growth and reproduction of healthy cells. Scientists believe that insulin imbalance has the potential to stimulate the growth of cancer cells.[5]

INFLAMMATION AND HORMONAL DEREGULATION

Inflammation and hormonal deregulation are among the main mechanisms linking excess weight to an increased cancer risk.

Extra body fat is associated with chronic inflammation. Even at low levels, continuous inflammation leads to reduced immunity, increased free radical production, and cell damage.

Increased body fat is a primary source of hormonal deregulation, mainly leading to high levels of estrogen production. Fat cells produce estrogen, leading to estrogen imbalance or dominance. Women with excess body fat tend to have higher levels of estrogen, which promotes the growth of estrogen-sensitive cancers such as endometrial and breast cancer.[6]

VITAMIN AND MINERAL DEFICIENCIES

Despite excessive food and calorie intake, many overweight people have deficiencies in vital nutrients. This is mainly because of the high availability of foods with "empty calories." This is a term used to describe processed foods that are high in calories and very often rich in sugar, white flour, and processed fats. Though these foods are high in calories, they lack essential vitamins like folate and other B-complex vitamins, antioxidant vitamins like C and E, and vital minerals such as magnesium and zinc, and therefore offer very little or no nutritional value.

Specific nutrient deficiencies lead to a compromised immune system, to an impaired ability to repair DNA, and to a deregulated metabolism. All of these, in turn, enable cancer cell growth and development and disable the body's ability to protect against cancer.

WE CAN ALL BE PART OF THE CHANGE

With the rising obesity rates globally and in particular among young children, it's becoming extremely important that we all become aware of the link between excess weight and cancer. As a global community we can all help to prevent as many cancer cases as possible.

Each one of us has a role to play in helping our loved ones maintain a healthy weight. We can help our parents, children or grandchildren, and other family and friends to enjoy healthy foods and move more. We also can be healthy role models for the people around us and inspire others to live a healthy and balanced lifestyle.

Maintaining a healthy weight may be the single most important factor that can protect against cancer. So making the necessary changes so that you and your loved ones can reach and maintain a healthy weight is more important than ever.

Suggestions:

- Prevent further weight gain if you are overweight
- Aim to reach and maintain a healthy weight by making positive and permanent changes in your diet and increasing exercise
- Responsibly teach healthy eating habits to your children in order to help them grow while maintaining a healthy weight and preventing childhood obesity

CHAPTER 4

The Importance of Weight after a Cancer Diagnosis

NOT ONLY IS EXCESS WEIGHT one of the main factors increasing the risk of developing cancer in the first place, it also plays a key role in the management of the disease.

WHAT DOES IT MEAN TO HAVE EXTRA WEIGHT AT THE TIME OF A CANCER DIAGNOSIS?

Obesity is generally associated with worsened outcomes following a cancer diagnosis.[1] More and more research is pointing out that obesity negatively affects the delivery of conventional cancer therapies such as chemotherapy and radiation, and reduces their efficacy.[2]

Having extra weight is also associated with more side effects resulting from common cancer treatments and more complications following surgical removal of tumors.

POSITIVE EFFECTS OF CONTROLLING WEIGHT AFTER BEING DIAGNOSED WITH CANCER

Overweight patients facing cancer can decrease the chance of cancer metastasis and increase the chances of treating cancer successfully by taking steps to lose weight.

Even a 5 to 10 percent decrease in weight can have significant improvements in the quality of life, physical fitness and psychology of people facing cancer.

It is also important to note that overweight cancer patients who lose weight generally maintain a better overall health status. They have better blood pressure and fewer risk factors for developing chronic diseases such as heart disease and diabetes.

A study published in 2014 in the journal *Gynecologic Oncology*, presented the results of a six-month lifestyle intervention program, offered to women with endometrial cancer. The women who participated in the intervention had achieved significant weight loss which was associated with improvements in their self-efficacy and overall quality of life.[3]

New research highlights the benefits of weight loss interventions for overweight and obese cancer patients. Overweight and obese cancer patients who participated in a fifteen-week-long healthy living program implemented through their oncology clinic lost an average of 4.6 kg. A control group from the same clinic who did not participate in the program gained 0.2 kg over the same period of time. The healthy living program focused on reducing calories by five hundred to one thousand per day and engaging in 150 minutes of moderate to intense exercise per week. Participants had an improved physical fitness at the end of the program and also reported improved sleep patterns and improvements in their fatigue levels.[4]

Other studies suggest that maintaining or increasing physical activity and controlling weight after a cancer diagnosis may improve the psychosocial well-being of breast cancer patients. In a study of 1,348 breast cancer patients, weight loss and maintenance was associated with less fatigue, depression, anxiety, and stress and better physical, social, emotional, and functional well-being.[5]

CAUSES OF WEIGHT GAIN DURING A CANCER TREATMENT

Many people gain weight after their treatments, especially for hormone-related cancers like prostate and breast cancer. Women whose treatment involves inducing menopause are the most likely to experience weight gain.

There are many factors that might contribute to weight gain with treatment of any cancer:

Fatigue is very common among people having chemotherapy and radiation, and can lead to less physical activity, which means fewer calories burned.

Nausea is another common side effect of these treatments, and many people eat frequent snacks to help deal with the nausea.

Some people eat more when they feel stressed out, and having cancer is by itself a very stressful situation that might lead to overeating.

Hormone changes or medications may cause people to feel hungry or retain water.

PREVENTING WEIGHT GAIN FOR PREVENTION OF CANCER RECURRENCE

According to the American Cancer Society, gaining weight after being diagnosed with cancer can give these patients a higher risk of the cancer returning.[6] In fact, a recent study showed that men who gained about five pounds (2.2 kg) in the years after surgery for prostate cancer had higher rates of recurrence than those with stable weight. For breast cancer, studies also suggest that weight gain after treatment can increase recurrence risk and decrease survival rate.

Suggestions:

- Assess your weight with your cancer care team.
- Discuss the effect your weight has on your overall health with your medical team and with a dietitian (preferably one that is specialized in cancer issues).
- Ask for help in achieving a healthier weight or in helping you to prevent weight gain during treatment.
- Follow a well-balanced diet and aim to achieve long-term improvements in your dietary habits.
- Add at least 150 minutes of moderate-intensity activity per week. Stay active to help combat fatigue and control side effects like constipation and nausea.

PART C

Vitamin D

CHAPTER 5

Vitamin D and cancer – A new Role for Vitamin D

DOCTORS HAVE TRADITIONALLY CONSIDERED vitamin D to be solely related to bone health, since it plays a central role in promoting calcium absorption. The scientific community has only recently begun to recognize the remarkable role of vitamin D in disease prevention and management. Nowadays vitamin D is considered to be a hormone rather than a vitamin, and it has been shown to play a central role in the healthy functioning of our bodies.

Various epidemiological studies have shown that as the levels of vitamin D in the blood increase, the incidence of major health problems, including heart attacks, diabetes, multiple sclerosis, and hypertension is reduced.[1] Conversely, low vitamin D levels have been shown to result in a malfunctioning immune system and to increase the risk of cancer.

According to Michael F. Holick, PhD, MD, who heads the Vitamin D, Skin, and Bone Research Laboratory at Boston University School of Medicine, activated vitamin D is one of the most potent inhibitors of cancer cell growth.[2]

Dr. Frank Garland and his brother, Cedric Garland, were the first to propose that vitamin D deficiency might contribute to a higher risk of cancer mortality, and specifically of colon cancer mortality.[3] They observed that breast and colon cancer mortality rates were twice as high in the US counties that had the least sunshine. This observation made them realize that there was a link between sunshine and cancer, and that link triggered their scientific interest. hey were the first to find an effect of oral intake of vitamin D on the risk of developing cancer.[4]

Thanks to their pioneering research, we now have numerous epidemiologic and laboratory studies showing an association between increased vitamin D in the blood and diet and a reduced cancer risk. Laboratory studies from the 1980s show that vitamin D inhibits the growth of malignant melanoma cells, leukemic cells, and skin cancer cells.

VITAMIN D IS REQUIRED FOR REGULATING NORMAL CELL GROWTH

Vitamin D is one of the most potent hormones for regulating normal cell growth. It was recently discovered that many different types of cells within the body contain vitamin D receptors. When these receptors are activated by vitamin D, the cells grow, function, and multiply in a healthy way. Vitamin D regulates normal cell growth by inhibiting abnormal development, invasiveness, uncontrolled angiogenesis, and metastatic potential.[5,6]

LOW VITAMIN D LEVELS ASSOCIATED WITH INCREASED CANCER RISK

Researchers on Vitamin D, including David Feldman, M.D., Professor of Medicine at Stanford University School of Medicine, have accumulated data from a large number of studies that strongly suggest that vitamin D deficiency increases the risk of developing cancer.[7]

The protective relationship between sufficient vitamin D in the body and lower risk of cancer has been found in many studies. A study by Frank and Cedric Garland back in 1989 found that low levels of vitamin D in the blood (below 20 ng/mL), were associated with a two-fold increase in the risk of developing colon cancer.[8] A similar study for colorectal cancer found that a blood level of vitamin D of 34 ng/mL can reduce the incidence of the disease by half, whereas a level of 46 ng/mL can reduce it by two-thirds.

VITAMIN D AND BREAST CANCER

Women with breast cancer are likely to have low levels of vitamin D in their body. Some research has shown that postmenopausal women who don't get adequate vitamin D may be more likely to develop breast cancer later in life. It has also been shown that women who have breast cancer are more likely to develop bigger tumors and are more likely to have recurrent breast cancer if they have low levels of vitamin D.

In a review of many studies, researchers found that among women with breast cancer who had low vitamin D levels, the risk of cancer recurrence was more than doubled, and the risk of mortality was almost doubled, compared to women with adequate vitamin D levels.[9]

A study done in 2009 in Canada followed a group of women with early-stage breast cancer over the course of twelve years. The study found that in women who have breast cancer, low levels of vitamin D are linked to worse outcomes, including bigger tumors and a higher risk of cancer spreading to other parts of the body.[10]

VITAMIN D REDUCES THE RISK OF METASTASIS

The reduced risk of metastasis in cancer patients with high serum vitamin D levels was also found in many other studies. Cancer patients with higher vitamin D levels were also found to live much longer than cancer patients with lower vitamin D levels.[11] Furthermore, vitamin D3 treatment significantly suppressed the viability of some cancers (for example, gastric cancer), and it has been proven that vitamin D3 can act synergistically with other anti-cancer drugs.[12]

CHAPTER 6

Optimize Your Vitamin D levels

VITAMIN D CAN BE OBTAINED through skin exposure to the sun, from our diet, and, if necessary, from supplements. Ultraviolet rays from the sun, specifically the UVB rays, trigger the production of vitamin D in the outer layer of the skin. This inactive vitamin D is then transported into the liver and the kidneys, where it is converted into its active hormone form, known as calcitriol.

The level of vitamin D in the blood is among the most important factors related to the risk of developing cancer and a wide variety of other diseases. Recent research has shown that for maximum health, vitamin D levels need to be at least between 40 and 60 ng/ml year-round.[1]

CAN YOU GET ENOUGH VITAMIN D THROUGH YOUR FOOD?

The vitamin D we get from food or supplements is measured in IU (international units). It can also be measured in micrograms (mcg or μg), and 1 mcg equals 40 IU.

Vitamin D is only found in a few foods. Fatty fish, fish liver oil, and eggs naturally contain vitamin D, but the amount of vitamin D in these foods is not enough to ensure a good vitamin D status. One egg yolk, for example, has an average of 50 IU of vitamin D. It is now believed that people who are not regularly exposed to the sun cannot get enough vitamin D from food alone.

HOW MUCH VITAMIN D IS NEEDED?

Different organizations recommend different daily Vitamin D intakes. An increasing number of researchers who specialize in vitamin D and cancer believe that taking low amounts, 1,000 IU or below, isn't enough, and suggest taking 2,000 to 5,000 IU of vitamin D3 per day.[2]

Aim for an intake of vitamin D that will keep your vitamin D levels at least between 40 and 60 ng/ml year-round. Doctors recommend that you check your vitamin D levels every six months, because it takes at least three months for it to stabilize after a change in sun exposure or supplement dose. Once you reach optimal levels it would be very wise to monitor your vitamin D blood levels regularly and start reducing your dose until you find the vitamin D supplement dose that keeps your vitamin D status at the desired range.

In people who are overweight, a large percentage of their vitamin D intake is stored in fat tissue, so they might need two to five times more vitamin D intake than lean people.

SAFE SUN EXPOSURE FOR OPTIMIZING VITAMIN D LEVELS

Sun-produced vitamin D is the most natural and efficient way to optimize the body's vitamin D levels. Exposing bare skin to the sun can quickly produce significant levels of vitamin D, especially in the summer, according to John J. Cannell, MD, founder and executive director of the Vitamin D Council.[3]

You don't need to tan or burn your skin to get vitamin D. According to the Vitamin D Council, you need to expose your skin for only around half the time it takes for your skin to turn pink and begin to burn.

Extra caution is needed, however, to build sun exposure slowly and to match your exposure to your skin type. Exceeding this safe level of sun exposure and letting the skin burn only causes damage to the skin and in the long run leads to an increased risk of skin cancer.

For most people, reducing cancer risk requires spending around twenty to thirty minutes in the sun every day.

FACTORS AFFECTING VITAMIN D PRODUCTION

When it comes to vitamin D production through sun exposure, the amount of skin you expose is obviously very important. The more skin your expose, the more vitamin D your body will produce.

According to the Vitamin D Council, the amount of vitamin D your body makes through exposing your bare skin to the sun depends on the following things:[4]

- The time of day: Your skin produces more vitamin D if you expose it during the middle of the day.

- Where you live: The closer to the equator you live, the easier it is for you to produce vitamin D from sunlight all year round. People living further away from the equator have fewer UVB rays available, particularly during the winter, so supplementation is necessary. For example, in cities like New York and Boston and in the Scandinavian countries, one cannot produce enough vitamin D through sun exposure from November to March.

- Your age: As you get older, your skin has a harder time producing vitamin D.
- Whether you're wearing sunscreen: Sunscreen blocks a lot of vitamin D production.
- The altitude you're at: The sun is more intense on top of a mountain than it is at the beach. This means you make more vitamin D at higher altitudes.
- The weather: Less UVB reaches your skin on a cloudy day, and therefore your skin makes less vitamin D on those days.
- Air pollution: Polluted air soaks up UVB or reflects it back into space. This means that if you live somewhere where there is lots of pollution, your skin makes less vitamin D.
- Being behind glass: Glass blocks all UVB, so you can't make vitamin D if your exposure to sunlight is from behind glass.

SKIN TYPE AND VITAMIN D PRODUCTION BY SUN EXPOSURE

Pale skin makes vitamin D more quickly than darker skin. Melanin, the substance that affects how light or dark your skin color is, affects the amount of vitamin D you can produce. Melanin protects against skin damage from too much UVB exposure. Darker skins have more melanin and allow less UVB to enter the skin. With less UVB getting through the skin, less vitamin D is produced each minute. This is why if you're dark skinned, you need more sun exposure to make vitamin D than if you're fair skinned.

If you have white or creamy white skin, are fair, and have red or blond hair and blue, green, or hazel-colored eyes, then you produce vitamin D more quickly than if you have a darker skin type. For example, very fair people with red or blond hair, blue eyes, and freckles might need around fifteen minutes of sun exposure to get the vitamin D they need. People with dark brown, Middle-Eastern skin types might need up to six times longer (up to two hours) to produce the same amount of vitamin D.

WHAT IF FOOD AND SUN ARE NOT ENOUGH?

You can also get vitamin D by taking supplements. This is a good way to get vitamin D if you don't have the opportunity to spend at least twenty to thirty minutes every day in the sun or if you're worried about exposing your skin.

Vitamin D3 is the bioactive form of the vitamin, so it is important to make sure you are supplementing with vitamin D3 and not with other forms of the vitamin like vitamin D2. It comes in a number of different forms, such as tablets, capsules, or liquid, and it doesn't matter what form you take. For most people vitamin D is easily absorbed in the body, so you don't need to worry about what time of day you take it or whether you take it with meals.

IF YOU TAKE VITAMIN D YOU NEED TO CONSIDER YOUR VITAMIN K2 LEVELS TOO

If you're taking vitamin D supplements, you need to consider your vitamin K2 levels. Vitamin K2 deficiency may lead to vitamin D toxicity, which causes inappropriate calcification, resulting in hardening of the arteries and promotion of heart disease and stroke.

According to Dr. Kate Rheaume-Bleue, a naturopathic physician and author of the book *Vitamin K2 and the Calcium Paradox*, lack of vitamin K2 increases the risk of osteoporosis, heart disease, and cancer.[5]

Vitamin K2 is important because it moves calcium around the body. It removes calcium from areas where it shouldn't be, such as in your arteries and soft tissues. Vitamin K2 can be found in fermented foods, such as sauerkraut, kefir, and traditional sheep's yogurt, and it can also be produced by beneficial bacteria in the gut.

The other main role of vitamin K2 is to activate proteins that control cell growth. According to Dr. Rheaume-Bleue, this means that vitamin K2 has an important role to play in cancer protection.

Suggestions:

- Check your vitamin D levels as part of your routine blood tests.
- Aim to keep your vitamin D levels at least between 40 and 60 ng/ml year-round.
- Especially in winter, you might want to use a vitamin D supplement to ensure adequate vitamin D levels.

Increase Consumption of the Foods that Fight Cancer

CHAPTER 7

Cancer Prevention through Food

THE WORLD HEALTH ORGANIZATION estimates that as many as 30 percent of all cancer cases are directly linked to poor dietary habits and are therefore preventable by changes in our diets. This potential for prevention can have a huge impact on minimizing the burden cancer poses today on our societies and on people's health.

Some cancers are affected even more by our diets. For example, it has been estimated that when it comes to cancers of the gastrointestinal tract, a much higher percentage, up to 70 percent of them, can be prevented by improving our diets alone.[1]

Adopting new dietary habits is a wise thing to do both to prevent cancer developing in the first place (primary prevention) and to reduce the risk of recurrence once you have completed your treatment (secondary prevention). Learning what is best to eat and drink and what is best to avoid will also help to speed up recovery during treatment.

Extensive research has shown that a well-nourished cancer patient can better manage the disease. Eating a nourishing diet and combining nutrients and herbs that work synergistically with each other and with other treatments are key components in the challenge of beating cancer.

The chapters that follow will guide you through fascinating research findings that prove that what we eat can have a profound effect on minimizing our cancer risk.

As more and more research on the field is being done, the recipe for cancer prevention appears more obvious than ever:

- Increase consumption of the protective foods proven to have potent anticancer properties.
- Decrease consumption of the "dangerous" foods known to create an internal environment that supports tumor growth and development.

FOODS THAT FIGHT CANCER

In the last few decades we have seen the identification and study of a great number of powerful superfoods, of phytonutrients in spices and herbs, and of natural food components that through a wide variety of mechanisms help the body rebalance, fight inflammation, stop cancer growth, reduce cancer risk, or even overcome cancer.

There is strong evidence that a diet filled with a variety of plant foods such as vegetables, fruits, whole grains, and beans helps lower the risk for many cancers. The evidence clearly shows that a carefully planned diet can rebalance one's physiology and reverse the conditions that nurture cancer cells.

We all fight cancerous cells numerous times in our lives. If our diets are rich in natural ingredients from a whole food diet, then powerful protective nutrients and phytonutrients help the body beat cancer. Quoting from the book *Foods to Fight Cancer* by Professor Richard Beliveau and Dr Denis Gingras, "preventing cancer through diet equals non-toxic chemotherapy, because it makes use of the anticancer molecules present in food. These molecules fight cancer at the source, before it can reach maturity".[2]

The research that is available today is suggesting that natural compounds found in everyday foods target cancer development at all stages, from cancer initiation to cancer promotion and progression:

- Some compounds act by protecting the DNA and preventing cancer initiation at its very first stages.
- Others act by blocking angiogenesis, the formation of new blood vessels that feed cancer cells.
- Certain dietary compounds reduce inflammation.
- Specific compounds show very selective toxicity against cancer cells, directly and specifically commanding them to commit suicide (apoptosis) while protecting the body's healthy cells.
- Some compounds enhance the body's natural detoxification systems.
- Others act synergistically with chemotherapy medications and increase their effectiveness.

The list of cancer-fighting foods is endless, ranging from berries to apples, from flaxseeds to Brazil nuts, from green leafy vegetables to broccoli, and from garlic to turmeric.

CHAPTER 8

Fruits and Vegetables

THE WORLD HEALTH ORGANIZATION has estimated that approximately 1.7 million deaths worldwide (2.8 percent of the total) are the result of too little fruit and vegetable consumption. Insufficient intake of fruit and vegetables is also estimated to cause as many as 14 percent of gastrointestinal cancer deaths.[1] These estimates show that there is a strong potential for cancer prevention by simply increasing fruit and vegetable consumption.

The International Agency for Research on Cancer (IARC), which is the specialized cancer agency of the World Health Organization, estimates that 5 to 12 percent of all cancers can be prevented by increasing fruit and vegetable intake in people's diets. Furthermore, they estimate that by increasing fruit and vegetable intake, up to 20 percent of the high gastrointestinal cancers (stomach and esophagus) can be prevented worldwide.[2]

The American Institute for Cancer Research recommends that all of our meals should be mainly based on plant foods including vegetables, fruits, whole grains, and legumes such as beans.[3] Research shows that vegetables and fruits have the capacity to protect against a range of cancers, including mouth, pharynx, larynx, esophagus, stomach, lung, pancreas, and prostate.

WHAT'S SO IMPORTANT ABOUT FRUITS AND VEGETABLES?

There are many reasons why vegetables and fruits reduce cancer risk. As well as containing vitamins and minerals, which help keep the body healthy and strengthen our immune system, they are also good sources of other substances like phytonutrients. Phytonutrients are plant chemicals that are biologically active compounds in the human body. They have been extensively studied and found to protect cells from damage that can lead to cancer.

PHYTONUTRIENTS

Phytonutrients are the molecules that give color and organoleptic properties to fruits, vegetables, and spices. By organoleptic properties we mean properties that affect the organs and senses, for example, the characteristic taste and odor of garlic and onions is due to their high content of sulphur-containing phytonutrients. Phytonutrients are emerging as the most important anticancer compounds in fruits and vegetables.

There are many types of phytonutrients found in fruits and vegetables. Polyphenols are the largest class, as more than four thousand polyphenols have been identified. They are found in large quantities in grapes, apples, onions, and most of the brightly colored fruits.

While some phytonutrients have a strong antioxidant capacity, their full anticancer potential is exerted through a variety of mechanisms that work against cancer initiation, promotion, and progression. Some of the most important anticancer phytonutrients include the ellagic acid found in berries, resveratrol which is found in grapes, sulforaphane which is found in broccoli and many others which will be analyzed extensively in the next chapters.

Fruits and vegetables are also great sources of fiber, which is directly linked to a reduced risk of cancer. The anticancer properties of dietary fiber will be analyzed in more detail in chapter 16. Vegetables should be making up at least half of our main meals, as they decrease the caloric density of meals and help in maintaining a healthy weight.

Fruits are the best snack options for people of all ages, as they are much lower in calories than other snack options and are not processed.

Suggestion:

- Eat two to three portions of fruit and three to seven portions of vegetables each day.

- A portion of fruit equals to one medium-sized apple, pear, orange, nectarine, banana, or two smaller fruits like mandarins, figs, prunes, kiwi and apricots. When it comes to even smaller fruits a portion equals to approximately seven or eight strawberries, twelve to fourteen cherries, fifteen grapes, or half a cup of pomegranate. A portion of larger fruits equals to half medium slice of watermelon, one average slice of melon, or half grapefruit. A portion of dried fruit is around thirty grams, which equals to one heaped tablespoon of raisins, currants or dried berries, one tablespoon of mixed fruit, two dried figs or three dried prunes.

- A portion of vegetables equals to two to three broccoli spears or four tablespoons of cooked kale, spinach, spring greens or green beans. When it comes to salad vegetables, one cup of leafy vegetables, one average carrot, one medium tomato or seven cherry tomatoes can count as one portion.

ACID / ALKALINE BALANCE

Another reason why fruits and vegetables may help protect against cancer is that they help in maintaining a healthy acid / alkaline balance.

The average Western diet is rich in acid-producing foods such as meat, poultry, fish, dairy products, white processed flour and grains, caffeine, sugar, soft drinks, and salt. The most alkaline-forming foods are fruits, vegetables and pulses. Compared to diets such as the traditional Mediterranean, Asiatic, and Indian diets, the average Western diet is low in fruit and vegetables, the main alkaline-producing foods.

Lab studies have shown that cancer cells thrive in an acidic environment and that they cannot survive in alkaline surroundings.[4]

The human body, however, has an amazing ability to monitor the blood pH closely and to maintain a steady pH in the blood. It naturally compensates and rebalances the acidic pH that results from acid-producing foods by activating its own buffering system. This system involves bicarbonate and phosphate (bicarbonate is alkaline) which are stored in the bones. This buffering system is crucial to the body and is responsible for keeping our blood pH (a measure of acidity) within a very narrow range (7.35–7.45).[5] This pH level is slightly alkaline.

Eating more alkaline foods does not make your blood alkaline, but it definitely makes it much easier for the body to maintain the ideal pH range. At the moment there is no scientific literature establishing the benefit of an alkaline diet for the prevention of cancer. [6]

If a person's body is under stress, however, due to dealing with a cancer or dealing with the side effects of common cancer treatments, then it is logical that choosing foods that don't put too much strain on the body for maintaining a stable pH will help the body rebalance more easily.

Suggestions:

- Avoid processed foods, sugar, and salt in order to make your diet more alkalizing.
- Limit animal protein to a few portions per week.
- Add more fruits and vegetables to your diet in order to make it easier for your body to maintain the ideal acid / alkaline balance.

CHAPTER 9

Antioxidants, Free Radicals, and Cancer

FREE RADICALS

Like most chronic diseases, cancer is caused in part by free radical damage. Free radicals are atoms or molecules that have lost one electron, leaving them with an unpaired electron.

The electrons that surround the nucleus of an atom are supposed to be paired, so free radicals become very unstable and start attacking surrounding molecules in order to "steal" electrons. When the "attacked" molecules lose their electrons, they become free radicals themselves, and a chain reaction begins.

Free radicals, also known as reactive oxygen species, are a major cause of injury in vital body molecules. They are known to damage the DNA, cell membranes, and various lipids and proteins in the body.[1]

Free radicals are created in the cells through normal metabolic processes. They can also be produced by external, environmental factors like extended UV light exposure, smoking, toxic chemicals in food and the water supply, contact with carcinogens, radiation, stress, pollution, and inflammatory processes.

ANTIOXIDANTS

Antioxidants are nature's way of defending cells against attack by free radicals, helping the body resist aging. The body can manufacture some antioxidants but not others. The body's natural antioxidant production tends to decline with age.

Antioxidants "neutralize" and block the damaging effects of free radicals and limit their effect on the cells. In other words, they convert free radicals into harmless by-products.

Insufficient levels of antioxidants and factors inhibiting the antioxidant enzymes cause what is known as "oxidative stress," which damages or kills cells. Oxidative stress is responsible for many human diseases, including cancer.

A diet rich in antioxidants has been shown to prevent and help in improving the progress of all chronic diseases, including cancer. Hundreds of antioxidant substances have been identified and studied extensively. Antioxidants from the diet include vitamins such as beta-carotene and vitamin C, co-enzymes (i.e., co-enzyme Q10), phytonutrients, and essential metals like zinc and selenium. In the last few decades very powerful antioxidants have been identified in fruits and vegetables that are not classified as vitamins and are widely known as phytonutrients.

ORAC: MEASURING THE ANTIOXIDANT CAPACITY OF FOODS

The capacity of a food to neutralize—that is, scavenge free radicals—can be measured in the ORAC scale, which has been created by the US Department of Agriculture. The Oxygen Radical Absorbance Capacity (ORAC) scale expresses in short the antioxidant capacity of each food.

WHY IS ORAC IMPORTANT?

An ORAC unit is defined as a measure of the ability of antioxidants to absorb oxygen free radicals in the body. The ORAC test integrates the strength and duration of antioxidant protection for a food or substance into a single numerical value. It has been shown to highly correlate with the level and the duration of protection in cells, body tissues, and blood levels.

ORAC is therefore important because it is an indication of a food's ability to provide the body and blood with immune-enhancing factors (antioxidants) that combat oxidizing (rusting) of the body's cells, membranes, and tissues. In other words, it reflects a food's anticancer and anti-aging potency.

The list below presents the fruits and vegetables with the highest ORAC values. Besides fruits and vegetables, some common herbs and spices, cocoa and dark chocolate also have incredibly high ORAC values.

FRUIT (100 gr.)	ORAC Value
Acai berry, freeze-dried	102,700
Goji berries	25,300
Elderberries, raw	14,697
Cranberries, raw	9,584
Currants	7,960
Blueberries	6,552
Prunes	6,552
Blackberries	5,347
Raspberries	4,882
Apples, red delicious	4,275
Strawberries	3,577
Figs	3,383
Cherries	3,365
Apricots, dried	3,234
Cabbage, red	3,145
Broccoli	3,083
Apples	3,082
Raisins	3,037
Pears	2,941
Blueberry juice	2,906

Suggestion:

Aim for an intake of around 6,000 ORAC units a day. Pick at least three options from the list below daily. Each food in the list contains approximately 2,000 units.

1. ½ teaspoon ground cinnamon
2. ½ teaspoon dried oregano
3. ½ teaspoon ground turmeric
4. 1 heaped teaspoon mustard
5. 1/5 cup blueberries
6. ½ pear or grapefruit or 1 plum
7. ½ cup of black currants, berries, raspberries, or strawberries
8. ½ cup cherries
9. 1 orange or 1 apple
10. 4 pieces of dark chocolate (70% cocoa)
11. 7 walnut halves
12. 8 pecan halves
13. ¼ cup pistachio nuts
14. ½ cup cooked lentils
15. 1 cup cooked kidney beans
16. 1/3 medium avocado
17. ½ cup red cabbage
18. 2 cups broccoli
19. 1 medium artichoke or 8 asparagus spears
20. Medium glass red wine

List created by Patrick Holford, founder of the Institute of Optimum Nutrition.[2]

BERRIES HAVE THE HIGHEST ANTIOXIDANT CAPACITY

Berries have long been known to stand out for their anticancer potential. They are effective in blocking both the initiation and progression stages of tumor development.

Berries are very rich in phytonutrients. Due to their exceptionally high content of phenolic and flavonoid compounds, berries exhibit a high antioxidant potential, much higher than many other foods.[3,4]

Berries are among the top listed foods in the ORAC scale.

The various antioxidants found in fruits like berries act synergistically, meaning that their protective capacity is multiplied when they coexist, so it's much better to eat the fruit rather than take a single supplement.

Through their ability to "mop" free radicals and reduce cell DNA damage, to stimulate antioxidant enzymes, and to enhance DNA repair, berry compounds have been shown to inhibit cancer initiation.[5]

Additionally, they inhibit cancer cells' progression by reducing the growth of pre-malignant cells, promoting cancer cell death, reducing tissue inflammation, and inhibiting the blood supply necessary for tumors to grow.[6]

There have been many laboratory and human studies demonstrating the protective effects of berries and berry constituents on oxidative and other processes leading to cancer development.

Berries may be the most beneficial fruits to eat for cancer prevention, according to scientists at the American Institute of Cancer Research: "Research is providing new evidence that berries not only contain strong antioxidants that help to prevent cell damage that precedes cancer: they also appear to affect genes that are associated with inflammation and the growth of cancer".[7]

BLUEBERRIES AND THEIR SPECIAL COLOR PIGMENTS

The fruits with the highest antioxidant levels are the ones with the deepest colors, such as blueberries, raspberries, and strawberries. Blueberries stand out among all other berries because they contain the highest amounts of the powerful antioxidants and flavonoids that help prevent cell damage.

North American Indians, the Chinese, and the Europeans all used blueberries in their traditional herbal medicines. Those medicines typically derived from the dried leaves, fruits, roots, and seeds and contained anthocyanins naturally present in the plant.

Today, researchers report that the anthocyanins in blueberries play a significant role in inhibiting inflammation and tumor growth and in counteracting oxidation, all processes that damage healthy cells.

Blueberries are particularly high in anthocyanins, the color pigments responsible for the berries' intense blue color. Eating foods rich in anthocyanins may play a role in preventing lifestyle-related diseases. It is now believed, however, that this protection arises from the interactions of all the food components and phytonutrients found in berries and not just from one particular molecule.

Blueberries are also an excellent source of vitamins C and K and manganese and are a good source of dietary fiber. Besides anthocyanins, they also contain catechins, quercetin, kaempferol, and other flavonoids, as well as ellagic acid and resveratrol.

ELLAGIC ACID: THE ANTICANCER COMPOUND IN BERRIES

The interest in berries as anticarcinogens began in the late 1980s, when Gary David Stoner, a cancer researcher, discovered that ellagic acid, found in many fruits and vegetables, inhibited the genesis of tumors. He then found that berries contained high amounts of ellagic acid, and that black raspberries in particular had more of this compound than any of the other berries.

Ellagic acid is a phytonutrient found in raspberries, strawberries, cranberries and pomegranates. This natural plant chemical is also found in walnuts and pecans and its role in nature is to protect these plants from germs, fungi, bugs, and other threats.

Research in laboratory animals has found that ellagic acid can slow the growth of tumors caused by certain carcinogens. It can act as a strong antioxidant and has been found to cause cell death in cancer cells in the laboratory. In other lab studies, ellagic acid was found to reduce the effect of estrogen in promoting growth of breast cancer cells in tissue cultures. Scientists report that it may also help the liver to break down or remove some cancer-causing substances from the blood, helping the body detoxify.[8,9,10]

GOJI BERRIES: A TRUE SUPERFOOD

Goji berries, also known as wolfberries or lycium fruit, are a member of the nightshade family, which contains many other common vegetables such as tomato, eggplant, and pepper. They are considered to be among the most nutritionally dense fruits on earth. Goji berries have gained huge popularity over the past decade because of their antioxidant properties.

Goji berries have been used for thousands of years in Tibet and China as an important part of traditional medicine and medical diets.

In the last decades a large number of lab and animal studies have been conducted with goji berries. From these studies we know that a number of natural components isolated from goji berries have multiple pharmacological properties, including antioxidant, anti-aging, immune boosting, and anticancer activity. They are also known to have blood pressure–lowering effects, to help in body fat reduction, and to protect hepatic function.[11,12]

Goji berries score among the highest ORAC values, compared to other fruit and vegetables. Goji berry juice was found to improve antioxidant biomarkers in healthy adults. This proves that the antioxidant molecules that give goji berries their high ORAC score are absorbed and utilized within the body.[13]

The two major active ingredients in goji berries, L. barbarum polysaccharides (LBP) and AA-2βG, a vitamin C analogue, were found in research to cause cancer cell death and to enhance the effects of other cancer therapies.[14]

Goji berries were shown to have synergistic actions with chemotherapy and radiation and to reduce their side effects.[15] Some examples of this synergistic action are found in animal studies. One such study showed that LBP from goji berries enhanced the effects of radiation on acute cells of lung cancer.[16] In another animal study, goji berries were found to reduce the toxic effects to the heart associated with the chemotherapy drug doxorubicin.[17] Another promising mechanism was shown in a third study, where goji berries inhibited the growth of estrogen receptor–positive breast cancer cells.[18]

Even though human data are limited at this moment, all of the above findings suggest that goji berries can be used to supplement our diets and that goji berries have a strong potential to act as an anticancer agent aiming at the prevention and potential treatment of cancer.

One cautionary note is that people who are taking anticoagulant therapy such as warfarin should avoid regular use and high doses of goji berries or goji juice. A few cases of elevated INR in patients on anticoagulant therapy were reported following consumption of concentrated Chinese herbal tea made from goji berries. INR is a blood test that checks how long it takes for blood to clot. The higher the INR, the longer it will take blood to clot (and the higher the risk of bleeding).

Suggestions:

- Eat four to five servings of berries per week. Fresh, dried or unsweetened frozen berries are all good choices. Try to combine different berry types, as they appear to act with different mechanisms.
- Eat Goji berries daily while receiving cancer treatments like chemotherapy and radiotherapy to enhance the effectiveness of the treatments and to reduce their toxic effects on healthy cells and tissues (but avoid if using anticoagulant therapy such as warfarin).

CHAPTER 10

Other Super Foods that Help Prevent Cancer

GRAPES

Grapes are one of the most ancient fruits in the world. They are very popular and are enjoyed throughout the world. They are considered to be among the healthiest and most easily accessible fruits. Surprisingly, grapes belong in the wider family of berry fruits.

Wine, the result of the fermentation of grape juice, has been produced for thousands of years. Apart from having a central role in celebrations and festivities in many cultures throughout the centuries, in many cases in history wine has been recommended for the treatment of ailments, even by the father of medicine, Hippocrates himself.

Grapes contain an overwhelming number of health-supportive phytonutrients. It is therefore not surprising that they have been shown to provide amazing benefits to many of our body systems and to be associated with increased longevity.

The health benefits of consuming grapes and red wine in moderate amounts include protecting the cardiovascular system, reducing inflammation, and helping in blood sugar regulation. Grapes are also known to have an extraordinary antioxidant capacity. Their antioxidant benefits lead to lower levels of free radicals in the body, less oxidative stress, and the protection of cell membranes.

Grapes and red wine have also been shown to be especially beneficial in cancer prevention.

RESVERATROL: THE PHYTONUTRIENT THAT PROTECTS GRAPES

Both grapes and grape juice are rich sources of resveratrol. Resveratrol is a recently discovered anticancer molecule that has received a lot of well-deserved attention for its health-protective and anti-aging properties.

Resveratrol belongs to a group of naturally occurring plant compounds known as salvestrols. Professor Dan Burke, one of the researchers who discovered salvestrols, has described them as "Probably the most significant breakthrough in nutrition since the discovery of vitamins."[1] Salvestrols are produced in plants as a way to protect themselves from attack by microorganisms such as parasitic fungus and bacteria and they are characterized by their bitter taste.

As might be expected, resveratrol is mainly found in the skin of the grapes in order to best protect them from disease. Red and purple grapes contain significantly more resveratrol than green grapes. Raisins have a relatively low level of resveratrol.

Unfortunately, research is now showing that salvestrols are severely depleted in modern food, as compared with the human diet of even a century ago. The introduction of modern intensive farming methods means that we now use disease-control spray programs on food crops that inhibit the natural production of salvestrols. In addition, salvestrols are being actively removed during food processing in order to improve the sweetness of products such as fruit juices. Moreover, modern crops are bred to be sweeter, so the salvestrol component in these newer varieties is being further depleted. Evidence indicates that salvestrols are disappearing from our diet at an alarming rate.

Red wine is a rich source of resveratrol, as it contains the skins of the grapes too. Drinking wine, however, cannot be considered to be a wise option for boosting one's intake of resveratrol, because recent expert reports have linked alcohol intake with cancer. More specifically, the American Institute for Cancer Research's second expert report presented strong evidence that alcohol is associated with increased risk for cancers of the mouth, pharynx and larynx, esophagus, breast, colon, and rectum.[2]

Salvestrols are also found in artichokes, asparagus, wild carrots, berries, and apples, but their levels vary greatly depending on the area and the variety. Resveratrol is also found in cocoa, dark chocolate, and peanuts. Organically grown fruits and vegetables tend to have higher salvestrol levels.

RESVERATROL: A PHYTONUTRIENT WITH STRONG ANTICANCER POTENTIAL

Resveratrol possesses strong antioxidant and anti-inflammatory properties.[3,4] Numerous laboratory and human studies have shown that resveratrol is also a potent anti-cancer phytonutrient. It has the ability to prevent the damage that triggers the cancer process in cells and tissues and to change various signaling pathways of the cancer cells.[5]

Resveratrol has been found to activate AMPK, a central energy biosensor within cells that plays a key role in the regulation of metabolism in response to changes in fuel availability. Activated AMPK leads to apoptosis (death) of colon cancer cells, leads chronic myelogenous leukemia cells to death, and enhances cancer cell response to radiation therapy.[6]

Extensive laboratory research points to resveratrol's ability to slow the growth of cancer cells and inhibit the formation of tumors in lymph, liver, stomach, and breast cells. In one series of studies, resveratrol blocked the development of skin, breast, and leukemia cancers at all three stages of the disease (initiation, promotion, and progression).[7]

Resveratrol is among the few natural polyphenolic compounds that have the capacity to bring about cancer cell death and to enhance the effects of standard cancer therapies. It is now being studied extensively in order to identify the best therapeutic strategies to incorporate its use.

From all of the above, it is clear that nature's pharmacy has a juicy and tasty super food to offer! Red grapes are not only delicious but also offer a powerful anti-cancer protection.

Suggestions:

- Since grapes are actually a type of berry, they fall within the general guideline of eating berries four to five times a week.
- Eat red and purple grapes daily when they are in season.
- Aim to include grapes or grape juice (one small glass a day) in your diet while receiving cancer treatments like chemotherapy and radiotherapy in order to enhance the effectiveness of those treatments.

- If you have diabetes make sure you count the carbohydrates in your grapes and adjust your insulin dose accordingly.

- If you have insulin resistance (centrally deposited extra weight, high blood sugars, high triglycerides and high blood pressure), aim to lose weight and stabilize your blood sugar before adding grapes and grape juice in your diet.

- Some alternative cancer centers suggest supplementation with high doses of food derived resveratrol while being on a cancer therapy program (near 2000 points per capsule). Even though this supplementation regime had positive results in a number of cancer cases, this is not yet backed up by enough scientific research.

- For the prevention of cancer you can enjoy the moderate consumption of red wine (two to three glasses per week) as part of a balanced diet such as the Mediterranean diet which is rich in fish, beans, fruit, vegetables and olive oil.

POMEGRANATE: A MEDITERRANEAN TREASURE

Pomegranate is a fruit that grows mainly in the Mediterranean and Middle East region. It has been shown to possess many medicinal properties, such as being a strong antioxidant and anti-inflammatory.[8,9] The name "pomegranate" comes from the Old French word for "seeded apple." Pomegranates and especially their juice are considered by experts to be extraordinary super foods, as they are packed with beneficial nutrients known to have health-protective and anticancer effects!

The antioxidant activity of pomegranate juice is three times higher than that of red wine and green tea.[10,11] Pomegranates owe their strong antioxidant activity to phytonutrients of the flavo-noids family, like anthocyanins, ellagic acid, and tannins.

Interestingly, the antioxidant activity appears to be higher in juices that are extracted from whole pomegranates than in juices obtained from the arils only.[12] All the compounds naturally found in pomegranate juice act in a chemical synergy. They are much more effective as a complete package in their anticancer activities than when tested in isolation as individual or purified ingredients.[13]

Pomegranates are also a great source of potassium and some B vitamins and have more vitamin C than oranges. They are a great source of fiber and they help in keeping the immune system in a top condition.

THE ANTICANCER POWER OF POMEGRANATE

The unique biochemical composition of the pomegranate fruit has recently drawn the attention of investigators, who are study-ing its exceptional healing qualities. Recent research has shown that pomegranate extracts selectively inhibit the growth of breast, prostate, colon, and lung cancer cells in laboratory studies.[14]

Researchers in Israel are pioneers in studying the protective effects of pomegranates. They believe that pomegranates have evolved a potent synergism and that nature has evolved an unu-sual plant that pushes all of the right mechanistic buttons to kill a cancer cell.

From animal and lab studies we know that the pomegranate's multilevel effect influences multiple cellular pathways and inhib-its cancer growth in a variety of ways. This synergistic effect in-hibits the creation of a tumor's blood supply and inhibits cancer cell growth. It also inhibits cancer cells' tendency to invade other tissues and even programs cancer cell death.[15]

POMEGRANATE AND PROSTATE CANCER

Human studies with natural protective foods and cancer are very limited. In 2006, some remarkable results were published by Allan Pantuck. Dr. Pantuck is a doctor and researcher at the University of California, Los Angeles (UCLA)'s Jonsson Comprehensive Cancer Center. Dr. Pantuck's team examined the effects of giving a glass of pomegranate juice per day to men with prostate cancer. The men who participated in the study had rising PSA levels after undergoing surgery or radiation. Pomegranate juice slowed the increase in blood levels of PSA.

PSA, or prostate-specific antigen, is a protein that is produced by the prostate gland and is found in the blood. It is routinely measured to estimate the growth and progression of prostate cancer. The time needed for PSA to double (PSA doubling time) is an indicator of the growth rate of prostate cancer. In cancer patients a short PSA doubling time can be translated to increased cancer growth, whereas a longer PSA doubling time is translated as a slower prostate cancer progression.

PSA doubling time in Dr. Pantuck's study increased from fifteen to fifty-four months. This is one of the very few studies to show the inhibition of cancer growth and cancer cell death as a result of a natural juice (pomegranate) in humans.[16]

Another study used capsules containing pomegranate juice extract in men with rising PSA levels after local therapy for prostate cancer. The pomegranate extract significantly increased the time needed for the PSA to double, which meant that cancer progression was inhibited. In both studies a relevant proportion of men even showed a decrease of PSA serum levels after consumption of pomegranate juice (15 percent and 13 percent, respectively).[17]

Unfortunately, in men with advanced prostate cancer, daily pomegranate juice consumption does not result in significant PSA declines compared to placebo.[18] We believe that the promising results with early prostate cancer will provoke more research with other cancer patient groups, in order to identify the best times, dosages, and the like for nutritional intervention.

Suggestions:

- Eat pomegranates daily when they are in season.
- Drink a glass of pure unsweetened pomegranate juice one to two times per week for the rest of the year.
- Men who are diagnosed with early-stage prostate cancer are advised to drink a glass of pomegranate juice daily or alternatively to take a daily capsule of pomegranate juice extract.

CRUCIFEROUS VEGETABLES

The term "cruciferous" refers to the family of vegetables that includes broccoli, cauliflower, Brussels sprouts, kale, cabbage, and bok choy. The family takes its name from the shape of their flowers, whose four petals resemble a cross. They are considered to be "the super-veggies," as the substances they contain are among the most important anticancer substances among all fruits and vegetables.[19]

High cruciferous vegetable consumption is linked to lower risk of several cancers, including breast, lung, prostate, and colorectal.

An observational study in Chinese women found that the highest intake of cruciferous vegetables cut the risk of developing breast cancer in half.[20] Other studies reported that eating cruciferous vegetables three times a week was associated with halving the risk of colon cancer and that high intakes of the same vegetables also reduced the risk of aggressive prostate and bladder cancer.[21]

PHYTONUTRIENTS IN CRUCIFEROUS VEGETABLES

This family of vegetables contains powerful phytonutrients known as glucosinolates. Glucosinolates work by releasing two classes of compounds, isothiocyanates and indoles that have an extremely high anticancer activity. In experimental studies these two compounds have been found to inhibit cancer growth and cancer cells' early development.[22]

The active anticancer compounds of the cruciferous vegetables are released when they are chewed. Chewing enables the mixing of the phytonutrients that are kept in some of the plant's cell compartments with enzymes present in other compartments. It is therefore better to chew your broccoli and cabbage well before swallowing, in order to maximize the release of these powerful phytonutrients and their availability for the whole body.

For optimum availability of the anticancer molecules avoid boiling these vegetables for long time periods in a large volume of water. Instead, try to use rapid cooking techniques such as steaming or stir-frying in a wok. If you are using water for cooking, use the minimum amount possible.

Fresh vegetables are considered to be superior to frozen ones, as they have higher amounts of glucosinolates.

SULFORAPHANE: A STRONG DETOXIFIER AND A STRONG CANCER WARRIOR

Sulforaphane was identified in 1992 as one of the strongest phyto-nutrients of the cruciferous family and has been extensively studied since then. The best source of sulforaphane is broccoli.

In lab studies, along with other phytonutrients found in cruciferous vegetables, sulforaphane was found to destroy many types of cancer cells by triggering apoptosis.[23]

Sulforaphane is particularly important in preventing cancer, as it enhances the body's ability to excrete carcinogenic substances. It has been shown to boost the effects of various detoxifying enzymes so that carcinogens are excreted before they damage cells.

Other studies have shown that the various compounds contained in cruciferous vegetables, and especially in broccoli, were able to prevent cancer cells from spreading to other parts of the body.

INDOLE-3-CARBINOL BLOCKS EXCESS ESTROGENS

Indole-3-carbonol (I3C) is another important anticancer phytonutrient. It is found in most cruciferous vegetables and especially in broccoli and Brussels sprouts. In recent research, I3C has proved to affect estrogen metabolism in a manner that blocks the development of estrogen-dependent cancers such as breast and uterine cancers.

OTHER PROTECTIVE NUTRIENTS IN CRUCIFEROUS VEGETABLES

Over the years, researchers have identified numerous substances in cruciferous vegetables that have shown anti-cancer potential.

Nearly all cruciferous vegetables are excellent or good sources of vitamin C, and some are good sources of manganese as well. Dark green vegetables are high in vitamin K. Other nutrients and phytonutrients in cruciferous vegetables vary:

Broccoli, Brussels sprouts, cauliflower, and rapini are all excellent sources of folate, a B vitamin that is involved in DNA synthesis and cancer prevention.

Broccoli, Brussels sprouts, and rapini contain carotenoids, such as beta-carotene.

Red cabbage and radishes also supply anthocyanins.

Other cruciferous vegetables provide different polyphenols, such as kaempferol and quercetin.[24]

Suggestions:

- Include cruciferous vegetables in your diet most days of the week.
- Choose broccoli and/or Brussels sprouts three to four times a week. Women at risk of estrogen-dependent cancers should focus more on broccoli and Brussels sprouts for their I3C content.
- Chew your cruciferous vegetables well. Use quick-cooking techniques such as steaming or stir-frying in a wok and use as little water as possible.

STONE FRUIT (PLUMS, PEACHES, AND OTHERS)

As scientists continue the research into natural compounds in the fight against cancer, new studies reveal that selected plums and red-fleshed peaches have antioxidant activity equal to or greater than that of blueberries. Scientists at the Texas AgriLife Research Lab found that breast cancer cells, even the most aggressive type, died after treatments with peach and plum extracts in lab tests, and not only did the cancerous cells die but the normal cells were not harmed at all.[25]

Peaches and plums belong to the "stone" fruit family and owe their anticancer activity to phenols, the compounds that occur naturally in fruits and are associated with the color, smell, and taste of specific fruits. Although these types of phenols are very common in fruits, stone fruits and especially plums and red-colored peaches are especially rich in them.

Peaches and nectarines, however, are also found on the list of the most contaminated fruits and vegetables as published by the Environmental Working Group. I would therefore advise that if it is possible, it is best to purchase organically grown forms of this fruit and purchase them only when they are in season.

Suggestions:

- Choose plums, peaches, and nectarines as your snack between meals when they are in season.
- If possible get organic to avoid the heavy contamination with pesticides.

MUSHROOMS HELP FIGHT CANCER

Until now we've all been adding mushrooms in our starters, main dishes, sauces etc in order to enjoy their unique texture, to boost the flavor of our dishes, and to create gourmet meals. As from now you will have another reason to use mushrooms frequently in your meals.

Mushrooms have long been used in traditional Eastern medicine; the earliest records go back over four thousand years in China. Like the Chinese, other nations from Japan to Korea and Taiwan have included the use of medicinal mushrooms in their treatment of many serious diseases, including cancer.

MUSHROOMS STIMULATE THE IMMUNE SYSTEM

Mushrooms contain compounds that have been linked to lowering the risk of a range of cancers. They have been found to stimulate the immune system by increasing the number and activity of our immune cells. Surprisingly, the anticancer effects of extracts of edible mushrooms were first reported back in 1969, in the journal *Cancer Research*.[26]

Since that time the anticancer activity of edible and medicinal mushrooms has been studied extensively. A meta-analysis of ten large studies on breast cancer, with a total of 6,890 cases, was published in 2014 by a team of Chinese researchers. They concluded that mushroom intake had protective effects against breast cancer in both pre- and postmenopausal women. The higher the mushroom intake, the greater was the level of protection. In their report, the scientific team concluded that polysaccharides present in mushrooms trigger a wide spectrum of host immune responses, which are capable of recognizing abnormal cancerous cells and eliminating them.[27]

In some studies, women who ate mushrooms had up to 50 percent lower risk of breast cancer compared to those who did not eat mushrooms.[28] Mushrooms are specifically effective in inhibiting the growth of estrogen-dependent breast cancers.

MUSHROOMS INCREASE SURVIVAL WHEN USED ALONG WITH CANCER TREATMENTS

Mushroom extracts are used along with chemotherapy and radiation in China and Japan. They have been found to reduce side effects of radiation and chemotherapy, including nausea and hair loss.

Patients with colorectal cancer who had surgical treatments for their cancers stayed in remission and were disease-free for a significantly longer period when given a mushroom extract. The people who received the mushroom extracts also lived longer.[29]

SHIITAKE, MAITAKE, ENOKITAKE, CREMINI, PORTOBELLO, AND OYSTER (OR PLEUROTUS) MUSHROOMS

With tens of thousands mushroom species around the world, it's only logical to wonder which are the ones that really stand out for their ability to deliver this tremendous boost to our immune system and which have been found to prevent and treat cancer.

Shiitake, maitake, enokitake, cremini, Portobello, and oyster (or pleurotus) mushrooms are the ones that are richer in the immune-enhancing compounds.

Cremini is actually one of the most widely consumed mushrooms in the world. It is actually the same common white mushroom that is very easily available in all Western countries, also known as the button mushroom or champignon. When it becomes more aged and brown it is known as a cremini, chestnut, or Italian mushroom. When mature, the same mushroom is known as the Portobello mushroom.

If you find oyster mushrooms on the market, remember that they are also known as pleurotus, and that they are the ones that in laboratory tests were shown to be the most effective against breast cancer cells.

Suggestions:

- Try to eat medicinal mushrooms twice a week.
- Choose shiitake, maitake, enokitake, cremini, Portobello, or oyster (or pleurotus), as they are richer in the immune-enhancing compounds.
- People doing chemotherapy or radiation can use mushroom extracts to enhance the treatment and reduce side effects.

GARLIC, ONION, LEEKS, CHIVES, AND SPRING ONIONS

Vegetables of the allium family include garlic, onion, leeks, chives, and spring onions. These vegetables are used all over the world in both simple everyday recipes and gourmet cooking. Throughout the years they also have been used medicinally for their antimicrobial, antibacterial, antithrombotic, immune system–boosting, lipid lowering, and blood glucose–lowering effects. In recent years their anticancer potential has been in the spotlight of scientific research.[30]

Epidemiological studies have shown that higher intake of the allium vegetables is associated with reduced risk of several types of cancers. These epidemiological findings are also backed by evidence from laboratory investigations. This family of vegetables is rich in sulfur compounds, which are capable of inducing death in cancer cells via a number of mechanisms. More specifically, these bioactive compounds have been shown to inhibit cancer development at the initial stages when changes in the DNA of normal cells lead to cancer. Furthermore, they have been found to neutralize free radicals and to inhibit tumor growth.[31]

Components of garlic extract (in combination or alone) have shown great potential in blocking angiogenesis (the formation of the blood vessels necessary for the survival of cancerous cells) and in preventing metastasis.

Suggestions:

- Add garlic to your meals as often as possible.
- Crush garlic, chop the onions, and dissolve in a little oil to make their bioactive compounds more readily available for absorption.
- Chop garlic, onions, and leeks, stir-fry them with a little olive oil, and use them to garnish steamed vegetables, rice, or any other dish. When raw, chopped garlic also can be added to good-quality butter from grass-fed animals or to olive oil.

SEAWEED: PROMISING ANTI-CANCER EFFECTS

In the last few years, a number of studies have explored the use of seaweed in the fight against several diseases, including colon and breast cancer.[32] Various therapeutic compounds from seaweeds have been identified as having promising effects against cancer. These compounds have been found to eradicate or slow the disease's progression.

One of these compounds is fucoidan, which is mainly found in various species of brown algae and brown seaweed such as kombu, also known as kelp, and wakame. Fucoidan was able to induce apoptosis, inhibit angiogenesis, and suppress metastasis of breast cancer in lab and animal studies.[33] Fucoidan contains antioxidants that protect against cell damage. The same compound can also combat inflammation and stimulate and balance the immune system.

A study published in April 2014 followed up on previous research showing that brown seaweed has a significant anti-estrogenic effect. The study identified the mechanisms involved in the anti-estrogenic activity of brown seaweed, which may prove to be particularly relevant in the pathogenesis and progression of female cancers such as breast cancer.[34]

Research on fucoidan is still at an early stage, so it is not possible at the moment to recommend a particular dose or a regular use of a supplement containing fucoidan. However, we would definitely recommend the incorporation of brown seaweed into a healthy diet, as has been done in Asian countries for thousands of years.

Suggestions:

- Add seaweed in your diet as often as possible.
- Most seaweeds are sold in their dried form. You can steam, sauté or boil dried seaweed to serve as a side dish or use in a recipe i.e. in salads, soups, noodle dishes etc.
- About 15 minutes is the time required to cook dried seaweed, no matter which method of cooking you choose.
- Once cooked, seaweed will keep for up to three days in the refrigerator, but is best used right away.

CHAPTER 11

Cancer Prevention through Herbs and Spices

HERBS AND SPICES

Herbs and spices have been used for thousands of years and are known for the flavor, taste, and color they add in foods. They have been used since ancient times not only to improve the flavor of food but also to prevent and treat disease. A great number of herbs and spices are nowadays being studied extensively for their medicinal powers and particularly for their anticancer effects.

TURMERIC

Turmeric is a yellow- to orange-colored spice that is part of the ginger family and is mainly imported from India. It is the spice that provides curry with its distinctive color and flavor.

The health benefits of turmeric have been recognized by practitioners of Chinese and Indian Ayurvedic traditional medicine for hundreds of years. Nowadays, many scientists consider turmeric to be a first-class super food.

Cancer rates in India are much lower than in Western countries. Indians have one-eighth as many lung cancers, one-ninth as many colon cancers, one-fifth as many breast cancers, and one-tenth as many kidney cancers, as compared to people of the same age living in the West.[1] Daily turmeric consumption is believed to play a key role in these huge differences in the rate of cancer development.

CURCUMIN

Over the last decade, numerous studies have explored the potential prophylactic or therapeutic value of curcumin, the bioactive natural compound in turmeric. Curcumin is a polyphenol with proven strong anti-inflammatory and antioxidant properties. It is believed that curcumin performs over 150 potentially therapeutic activities within the body. Extensive research has shown that curcumin has the ability to protect liver function, prevent thrombosis, and protect the heart. Curcumin is also used for treating arthritis, Alzheimer's disease, and, most importantly, cancer.[2]

Curcumin is the Golden Spice from Indian saffron, as characterized by Professor Bharat Aggarwal, head of the lab working on experimental cancer therapies at the M.D. Anderson Cancer Center in Houston. Professor Aggarwal is a pioneer cancer researcher who strongly believes in and extensively studies the anticancer effects of curcumin. He was the first to show that curcumin is very active against cancer in lab settings.

Since that time, curcumin has been studied extensively, and we now have enough scientific data from lab and animal studies to show that curcumin kills cancer cells and slows tumor growth.[3]

Curcumin acts on hundreds of cellular pathways and appears to be active on just about every type of cancer. More specifically, curcumin has been found to do all of the following things:[4,5]

1. Inhibit the reproduction of cancerous cells
2. Decrease inflammation
3. Inhibit the transition of cells from normal to cancerous cells
4. Inhibit the synthesis of NF-κB, which is a protein thought to play a key role in cancer formation, as it protects cancer cells from the immune system and allows their survival
5. Help the body destroy cancerous cells so that they cannot spread throughout the body
6. Help prevent the development of the additional blood supply necessary for cancer cell growth (angiogenesis).

Another discovery regarding curcumin that is extremely important is its ability to sensitize many human cancers to chemotherapy and radiation, including cancers that have been considered to be resistant to therapy.[6] The use of a curcumin-based, anticancer therapeutic strategy in the future will hopefully allow the use of lower doses of chemotherapeutic drugs and radiation with much greater anticancer results.

In animal models, curcumin was found to be very effective in protecting normal cells from the toxic effects of chemotherapy and radiotherapy. This lowered toxicity and enhanced protection was seen in a number of body systems, as curcumin was effective in preventing nephrotoxicity (toxicity of the kidneys), preventing oral mucositis, and reducing intestinal damage. Curcumin also enhanced the repair of wounds in mice exposed to whole-body radiation.

Curcumin is a safe and highly effective compound that can be used both in the prevention of cancer and also alongside the standard cancer therapies.

According to the conclusions of A. Goel and B. Aggarwal in an article published in the journal *Nutrition and Cancer* in 2010,

"Curcumin therapy may stop cancers before they become invasive and metastatic. These effects combined with its ability to prevent depression, fatigue, neuropathic pain, lack of sleep, and lack of appetite, all symptoms induced by cancer and cancer treatment, makes curcumin an ideal agent for cancer patients".[7]

Suggestions:

- Add turmeric to your meals as a flavoring in rice, salad dressings, soups, and other dishes.
- Add a pinch of black pepper to these dishes to aid turmeric absorption by the body.
- Tips for using turmeric in your recipes: mix 1 teaspoon turmeric powder with 1 tablespoon olive oil and a generous pinch of black pepper. Add to vegetables, soups, rice dishes, and salad dressings.[8]
- Curcumin supplements can be used by people suffering from chronic inflammatory conditions such as ulcerative colitis and Crohn's disease. The anti-inflammatory effects of curcumin are well established and may play a significant role in reducing the risk of developing colon cancer.

INCREASING CURCUMIN ABSORPTION

Curcumin is unfortunately very poorly absorbed in the human body, and the doses used for animal studies cannot be easily achieved by supplementation. However, traditional wisdom again shows us the way. In traditional Indian cooking, curry is mixed with pepper or ginger, substances that greatly boost absorption from our intestinal walls through the blood.

Mixing turmeric with black pepper and dissolving it in oil, preferably olive oil or linseed oil, greatly increases curcumin absorption.

GREEN TEA

Tea is the second-most consumed beverage worldwide after water. All tea is produced from the leaves of the plant *Camellia sinensis*, with different types of tea resulting from differences in the method of the leaves' processing. In the production of green tea, fresh tea leaves are steamed or heated immediately after harvest, resulting in minimal oxidation of the naturally occurring polyphenols in the tea leaves.[9]

High-quality tea has numerous health benefits. It plays a role in maintaining a healthy circulatory system and protecting against heart disease. It is full of antioxidants and detoxifies the body. It also possesses compounds with many anticancer properties.

The protective role of green tea against cancer is supported by a large number of laboratory and animal studies.[10,11] A great number of scientists have studied the activity of the major tea polyphenols, mostly catechins such as EGCG, EGC, and epicatechin. Polyphenols from tea are powerful antioxidants that also play a role in several mechanisms that could inhibit the initiation and progression of cancer.[12,13]

EGCG, epigallocatechin gallate, the most abundant catechin in green tea, may reduce DNA damage by reactive oxygen species and inhibit tumor cell growth, invasion, and angiogenesis. Adding to this, evidence from animal studies for several organ sites, including the esophagus, stomach, liver, colon, and pancreas, has shown that tea polyphenols and tea constituents inhibit tumor formation and cancer-promotional cellular mechanisms such as cellular proliferation, invasion, and angiogenesis.[14]

Despite the above data that show a protective role for green tea in cancer, however, results from human studies (prospective and epidemiological) have been promising but not consistent. Epidemiological studies compare the habits of large populations of people and study how they affect the risk of developing cancer or another disease. These studies suggest that drinking tea offers some protection against the development of cancer at several organ sites in humans.

In 2012, the results of a large prospective study were published in the *American Journal of Clinical Nutrition*.[15] This was a very large study that evaluated the effects of drinking tea (mainly green tea) in a total of 74,941 Chinese women aged forty to seventy years. This large and well-conducted study concluded that green tea consumption was associated with reduced risk of cancers of the digestive system, particularly cancers of the stomach, esophagus, and colorectum, in women. The women who consumed two to three cups of green tea per day had a 21 percent reduced risk of digestive system cancers. The reduction in risk increased as the amount and years of tea consumption increased.

In 2014 a great breakthrough was achieved in understanding the mechanism by which green tea can induce its anticancer activities. Dr.Qing-Yi Lu and his colleagues from the Department of Medicine of the University of California, Los Angeles, showed for the first time that treatment with EGCG, the major biological active constituent of green tea, inhibits the action of an enzyme that is essential in cancer cells' metabolism.[16] This enzyme, LDHA, controls the energy that enters the metabolic pathways of cancer cells. With the resulting inhibition of this enzyme, cancer cell survival and metastasis are both blocked and the body's natural immune response against cancer is optimized. The researchers noted that this study opens the door to a whole new area of cancer research and will help us understand how other foods can prevent cancer or slow the growth of cancerous cells.

Furthermore, even if the above research cannot prove the protective effects of green tea against cancer in an absolute way, we do know for sure that drinking green tea regularly does not cause any harm. In our opinion, drinking green tea daily does give your body a desired level of extra protection by robbing the cancer cells of energy, making metastasis more difficult and making the cancer easier to treat.[17]

Quoting the words of Dr. Joshua Lambert, a collaborator at the American Institute of Cancer Research, "Green tea would not necessarily be used as a front-line or single therapy, but perhaps as an adjunct to something else. . . . Green tea is most likely to be effective when used with another treatment for early-stage cancer or after chemotherapy treatment to prevent a recurrence".[18]

HOW HOT DO YOU LIKE YOUR TEA?

How can you make sure that the temperature of your tea is not canceling out its healthy benefits?

A study looking at the temperature of tea found that drinking steaming hot tea was linked with an increased risk of esophageal cancer. Drinking tea two to three minutes after pouring or less than two minutes after pouring was associated with a significantly increased risk compared with drinking tea four or more minutes after it was poured.

Compared with drinking warm or lukewarm tea, drinking hot tea (65 to 69 degrees Celsius) was associated with twice the risk of esophageal cancer, and drinking very hot tea (70 degrees Celsius or more) was associated with an eight-fold increase in risk.[19]

These results are similar to the results of a study that was published nearly a decade ago and found similarly that drinking hot beverages raise your risk of esophageal cancer by as much as four times. It is the temperature of the liquid that appears to be a problem and not the beverage itself.[20]

With this in mind, be sure to let your tea cool off a bit or add one or two ice cubes before you drink it.

MATCHA GREEN TEA

Matcha green tea is considered to be an antioxidant powerhouse. One cup of matcha green tea has the antioxidant power of ten cups of ordinary green tea. Matcha green tea possesses almost six times the antioxidant power of goji berries, seven times the antioxidant powers of dark chocolate, seventeen times that of wild blueberries, and sixty times that of spinach.

Matcha is a tea made from powdered green tea leaves that are mixed with water to create a green-colored tea. This means that you actually take in 100 percent of the green tea's unique nutrients, rather than just infusing your leaves and throwing away a lot of their goodness.

This is the original medicinal form of green tea. It was first introduced to Japan from China by Buddhist monks. Nowadays it is the most potent tea you can find.

Matcha tea contains L-theanine, an amino acid that promotes relaxation and has calming effects in the body. Zen Buddhist monks used to drink matcha tea to help them stay alert and calm during their long hours of meditation. The properties of matcha green tea are especially important in people living busy and stressful lives. Cancer patients would benefit from the calming effects of matcha green tea.

Caution: Green tea interferes with the chemotherapy drug bortezomib (Velcade) and other boronic acid–based proteasome inhibitors and therefore should be avoided by people taking these medications.[21]

Suggestions:

- Include green tea in your diet as often as possible.
- Aim to have two to three cups of green tea per day.
- Avoid drinking your green tea at a very high temperature.

THE POWERFUL ANTIOXIDANT ACTIVITY OF CULINARY HERBS

Recently herbs have been identified as sources of a variety of phytonutrients, many of which have strong antioxidant properties. In a study published in the *Journal of Nutrition* in 2003, a team from Norway and Japan assessed the contribution of culinary and medicinal herbs to the total intake of dietary antioxidants. They concluded that all of the dried culinary herbs tested (oregano, sage, peppermint, garden thyme, lemon balm, clove, allspice, cinnamon, and the Chinese medicinal herbs Cinnamomi cortex and Scutellariae radix) contained very high concentrations of antioxidants. They proposed that in a normal diet, intake of herbs may contribute significantly to the total intake of antioxidants. Herbs may even be a better source of dietary antioxidants than many such food groups as fruits, berries, and vegetables.[22]

Ground cloves, sumac, Ceylon cinnamon, and oregano have the highest ORAC values. The first two have an ORAC value of around 310,000 and the last two around 200,000. Ground turmeric scores around 100,000 ORAC units, which is equal to the very powerful antioxidant freeze-dried acai berry. Cocoa powder follows with an also high score of 80,000, together with cumin seed. Dried parsley and basil come next, with ORAC values around 70,000.

Hundreds of natural bioactive compounds have been identified from tested medicinal herbs. Their physiological and pharmacological functions originate from both their antioxidant and free radical–neutralizing properties and their ability to regulate detoxifying enzymes within the body.

CULINARY HERBS AND CANCER

It is worth noting that most drugs used for chemotherapy today are molecules identified and isolated from plants or their synthetic derivatives.[23,24]

A team of researchers from Israel studied whole-plant extracts from oregano, from the membranous nettle, and from artemesia. They found all three of them to be very effective in killing human cancer cells in lab tests. The lethal activity was induced by apoptosis (the mechanism forcing cancer cells to commit suicide). The higher the dose of the herbs, the higher was their effect in inducing cancer cell death. This activity was very specific to cancer cells, as the extracts had no effect on healthy human cells.

The culinary herbs peppermint, rosemary, sage, spearmint, and thyme extracts inhibit the growth of human colorectal cancer cells.[25] The herbs rosemary, sage, parsley, and oregano were also shown to be associated with reduced incidence of lung cancer.[26] Researchers have studied and identified the active compounds in these medicinal herbs. A specific phytonutrient named carnosol was identified and evaluated for its anticancer properties in prostate, breast, skin, leukemia, and colon cancer with promising results. Carnosol is a powerful antioxidant, and it targets numerous pathways associated with inflammation and cancer. In addition, carnosol has been shown to enhance the effectiveness of certain chemotherapies, where it shows a selective toxicity toward cancer cells versus healthy cells.

Although herbs and spices have always been used to improve the taste and color of food, it appears that they also have a key role in the prevention and treatment of a wide variety of chronic inflammatory diseases, including cancer.[27]

Suggestion:

- Use herbs and spices extensively in your cooking, as they do have a strong anticancer potential.

CHAPTER 12

Enzymes in the Fight against Cancer

ENZYMES SERVE A WIDE VARIETY of functions inside the body. Among other things, they are essential for cell regulation, digestion and metabolism. Enzymes such as amylases and proteases break down large molecules of nutrients such as starch or proteins into smaller ones, so they can be absorbed by the intestines and enter the bloodstream. Different enzymes digest different food substances.

BROMELAIN: A NATURAL ENZYME FOUND IN PINEAPPLE

Bromelain is a natural enzyme found in the stem and fruit of pineapples. Pineapples have been used for hundreds of years in traditional medicine as a digestive aid and to treat inflammation and other health problems.

In recent years, studies have shown that bromelain, the main bioactive compound of pineapple, has the capacity to act on key pathways that lead to carcinogenesis.[1]

Bromelain is a mixture of enzymes that break down proteins. It has recently been proven that when we supplement with bromelain, bromelain escapes digestion in the stomach, crosses the intestinal barrier, and enters the blood.

Once bromelain enters the circulation, it directly impacts cancer cells and their microenvironment. It boosts the immune system, reduces inflammation, and changes the hemostatic systems in ways that can enhance anticancer therapy. In animal, lab, and human studies, it has been shown that bromelain can inhibit cancer growth, lead to cancer cell death, and reduce metastasis.[2,3]

A proposed mechanism for the effectiveness of bromelain and other digestive enzymes in the treatment of cancer is that tumors have a protective protein layer that allows them to hide from the immune system and often offers them chemoresistance (resistance to therapy). This protein is known as MUC1 and is a glycosylation-dependent protein. Bromelain and other digestive enzymes can break down glycosidic bonds and therefore destroy the protective layer on the tumors, making them accessible to the immune cells.

A study published in 2010 found that long-term intake of pineapple juice inhibited the development of inflammation-associated colon cancers by decreasing inflammation.[4] The study involved an animal model of chronic colitis as seen in the very common inflammatory bowel disease.

In 2007 researchers published a groundbreaking article in the *Planta Medica* journal about bromelain. Their study found bromelain to be more effective than 5-fluoracil, a traditional chemotherapy medication used in the treatment of cancer. 5-fluoracil kills or irreversibly damages healthy cells and tissue along with the cancerous ones. Bromelain was not only found to be more effective but was also many times safer than 5-FU.[5]

In another study published in 2014 it was shown that in some types of cancer bromelain treatment was able to increase the effectiveness of another common chemotherapy drug, cisplatin.[6]

USING BROMELAIN

Bromelain is typically extracted from pineapples and packaged into capsule or tablet form.

When used as a digestive aid (if there is indigestion and malabsorption while on a chemotherapy program), bromelain supplements are usually taken with meals. The German Commission E, a scientific advisory board that is the German equivalent of the FDA, recommends 500 mg per day in divided doses with meals.[7]

When used for inflammatory conditions such as ulcerative colitis or when we need a systemic effect for inhibiting cancer growth and metastasis, doctors typically recommend that patients take bromelain between meals on an empty stomach to maximize absorption.[8]

Caution: People taking blood thinners (anticoagulant or anti-platelet medication, such as aspirin, warfarin [Coumadin], heparin, clopidogrel [Plavix], and nonsteroidal anti-inflammatory medications such as ibuprofen [Motrin, Advil] and naproxen [Naprosyn, Aleve]) should use bromelain only under a physician's supervision. Bromelain should also be used with caution by people taking herbs and supplements that are thought to increase the risk of bleeding, such as ginkgo biloba and garlic.

Suggestions:

- If you are simply looking to boost your immune system and help in the prevention of cancer, regularly drinking a glass of fresh pineapple juice seems to be the thing to do!

- If you feel you have indigestion take bromelain supplements with your meals. The German Commission E recommends 500 mg per day in divided doses with meals.
- If you would like to use bromelain together with other cancer treatments discuss it with your health care team and seek advice from a doctor specializing in naturopathic medicine.

CHAPTER 13

The Role of Good Fats in Cancer Prevention

THE BODY NEEDS FAT ON A DAILY BASIS. Healthy fats in the diet are vital for our survival and for the proper functioning of the brain, for membrane stability, for optimal heart health, for hormone production and reproduction, and even for the prevention of cancer.

THE MEDITERRANEAN DIET PROTECTS AGAINST CANCER

The Mediterranean diet is associated with a reduced risk of cardiovascular disease and cancer and has been proposed as a protective choice for cancer prevention.[1] Dr. Antonia Trichopoulou, M.D., Ph.D., Professor of Preventative Medicine and Nutrition at the University of Athens Medical School, published some promising and exciting estimations that up to 25 percent of colorectal cancer, 15 percent of breast cancer, and 10 percent of prostate, pancreas, and endometrial cancer could be prevented if people in developed Western countries would shift to the traditional healthy Mediterranean diet.[2]

The cancer-prevention effect of the Mediterranean diet is partly related to a balanced ratio of omega-6 and omega-3 essential fatty acids.[3] These fatty acids are essential because they cannot be synthesized in the body and need to be supplied from our diet.

OMEGA-6 TO OMEGA-3 RATIO, CHRONIC INFLAMMATION, AND CANCER

Omega-6 and omega-3 fatty acids are polyunsaturated fatty acids. They are lipids which are structurally different between them, and between saturated fatty acids. Their main characteristic is that they have many double bonds in their chain.

Our bodies work best when these two fats are in balance. We need to consume similar amounts of omega-6 and omega-3 fats. A ratio of 2:1 or 3:1 is considered ideal, however, most people eating a Western diet consume much higher amounts of omega-6 fats than omega-3, ranging from fifteen to thirty times more (15:1 to 30:1)!

The omega-3 fatty acids have a strong anti-inflammatory effect, whereas omega-6 fatty acids promote inflammation. Although inflammation is part of our body's defense system, chronic and sustained inflammation leads to the overproduction of free radicals, which cause DNA damage, activation of carcinogenesis, and inactivation of the ability to repair genes.[4] Chronic inflammation is strongly associated with various aspects of tumor promotion and spread, including effects on angiogenesis, immune function, glucose utilization, and apoptosis.[5,6,7]

Omega-3 fatty acids can lower cancer risk in various ways.[8] They suppress inflammation and diminish oxidative stress. They inhibit the production of blood vessels that feed tumors, inhibit tumor cell progression, and slow tumor growth. They are also involved in controlling the overproduction of estrogens, therefore reducing the estrogen-induced growth of breast cancer.[9] In addition, omega-3 fatty acids were found to prevent muscle wasting (cachexia) in cancer patients and to enhance the effects of certain types of chemotherapy and radiation treatments.[10]

Studies have also shown that a high blood level of omega-3 fatty acids combined with a low level of omega-6 acids reduces the risk of developing breast and prostate cancer.[11] Proving their potential for prevention, a daily supplementation with as little as 2.5 grams of fish oils (a rich source of omega-3 fatty acids) has been found effective in preventing the progression of benign polyps to colon cancer. Fish oil supplements have also been found to suppress metastasis and to improve survival and quality of life in very ill cancer patients.

FISH INTAKE REDUCES CANCER RISK

A summary of studies conducted in northern Italy found that people who consumed fish at least twice per week had a significantly lower risk for developing cancer compared to those who ate fish less than once a week. The cancers studied included cancer of the ovaries, endometrium, pharynx, esophagus, stomach, colon, and pancreas.[11] A similar Swedish study found that women eating two or more servings of fatty fish per week had a significantly lower risk for endometrial cancer.[12]

In 2012 a Chinese review article summarizing the results of forty-one studies found fish intake to have a strong protective effect against colon cancer.[13] Similarly, in a Polish study from

2008 focusing on colorectal cancer, fish intake offered a significant protection in people eating fish one to two times a week. The protection was even higher when fish intake was more than two times per week.[14]

With regard to breast cancer risk, high fish consumption was associated with a significant reduction in both premenopausal and postmenopausal women.[15]

Another great finding of recent studies is that a high intake, greater than three times per week, or the use of fish oil supplements, had the ability to decrease the incidence of metastasis.[16,17]

OILY FISH: OPTIMISING YOUR OMEGA-3'S

So, you now know that fish is good for you and that some fish are more beneficial than others. Fatty fish are the best sources of EPA and DHA, the longer-chained omega-3's, which are related to all the health benefits. Fatty fish are also protective against heart disease, arthritis, diabetes, and even depression. EPA and DHA are also found in the meat and dairy products of animals that are grass-fed.

It is very important to also note that farmed fish such as farmed salmon tend to have a higher omega-6 to omega-3 ratio than wild fish, as they are often fed with grains.[18,19,20] The long-chain omega-3's in fish are not synthesized by their digestive system but rather originate from microorganisms such as krill, at the base of their natural food chain. It is therefore preferable to eat more wild caught fish when it is available.

ANIMAL SOURCES OF OMEGA-3 ESSENTIAL FATTY ACIDS [21]

Fish (100 gr.)	Amount of omega-3
Sardines *	1080 mg
Anchovies *	2100 mg
Salmon - farmed **	2230 mg
Salmon – wild	1545 mg
Freshwater trout	1065 mg
Tuna	1457 mg
Mackerel	2800 mg
Herring	1564 mg
Farmed seabass	1700 mg
Farmed sea bream	2250 mg
Milk from grass-fed cows	500 ml milk = approximately 191 mg ALA and 14 mg EPA[22]

* Smaller fish have lower levels of mercury, compared to larger fish such as salmon and tuna.

** Farmed salmon from the Atlantic or from Scandinavian countries has recently been found to have higher than the allowed European levels of toxic PCBs and dioxins, so caution should be applied not to eat it frequently. Wild Alaskan salmon has less mercury than bigger fish like tuna and fewer PCBs than farmed salmon.[23]

CAUTION WITH FISH COOKING
AND PRESERVATION

Salted and preserved fish contain nitrosamines that are known to increase cancer risk, so these kinds of fish should be excluded. Frying fish significantly increases the omega-6 to omega-3 ratio, especially when using an omega-6-rich oil. Frying and other high-temperature methods of cooking fish, such as grilling and barbequing, also leads to the formation of heterocyclic amines and other chemicals that damage the DNA, so it's best to use other methods of cooking such as steaming and slow roasting.[24]

GRASS-FED ANIMALS HAVE SIGNIFICANTLY
HIGHER OMEGA-3 LEVELS

Research spanning three decades supports the fact that grass-fed beef is higher in omega-3 fatty acids and contributes to a better omega-6 to omega-3 ratio. It has a higher level of conjugated linolenic acid, a group of fatty acids that are associated with significant health benefits, including inhibition of carcinogenesis and reduction in body fat. Grass-fed beef is higher in precursors for Vitamin A and E and higher in cancer-fighting antioxidants as compared to grain-fed beef. Grass-fed beef also tends to be lower in overall fat content and is generally considered to be of much better nutritional quality.[25]

OMEGA-3 IN PLANT FOODS

Omega-3's are also found in some plant foods, such as flaxseeds, chia seeds, walnuts, and green, leafy vegetables. However, simply obtaining omega-3's from plants such as flaxseed or walnuts is unlikely to have a major impact on preventing cancer or metastasis or on the other health benefits of the longer-chained EPA and DHA. The reason for this is that the omega-3 fatty acid in plants, the alpha-linolenic acid, is a shorter-chained fatty acid that cannot be efficiently converted to the health-promoting EPA and DHA in the body.[26,27]

Keep in mind that it's the ratio of omega-6 to omega-3 that is important, so adding omega-3's from plants is still important for ensuring a good balance. In order to achieve the optimum ratio of 2:1 or 3:1, you must also keep your intake of omega-6 fatty acids as low as possible (omega-6 fatty acids and their sources are analyzed in the following chapters).

PLANT SOURCES OF OMEGA-3 ESSENTIAL FATTY ACIDS:[28]

Flaxseeds (28 gr)	6388 mg
Chia seeds (28 gr.)	4915 mg
Walnuts (28 gr)	2542 mg

Suggestions:

- Eat 120 to 150 grams of fatty fish two to three times a week.
- If possible, choose meat and dairy products from grass-fed animals, as they contain EPA and DHA.
- Avoid omega-6-rich oils to maintain a good balance of omega-3 to omega-6.
- Add chia seeds and grated flaxseeds to your muesli, salads, yogurt, and other recipes and use walnuts as a midday snack a few times per week.

FLAXSEEDS

Flaxseeds are associated with many health benefits, mostly attributed to their high fiber and omega-3 content. Flaxseeds also contain lignans, a class of phytoestrogens considered to have hormone-modulating effects, to act as antioxidants, and to possess cancer-preventing properties. Whole flaxseeds are commonly used to improve digestive health or relieve constipation. Flaxseed may also help lower total blood cholesterol and low-density lipoprotein (LDL, or "bad") cholesterol levels, a reduction that is related to a reduced risk of heart disease.

A group of researchers and practitioners from the Canadian College of Naturopathic Medicine and the Ottawa Integrative Cancer Center in Canada reviewed a number of studies on flaxseed and breast cancer. The scientific evidence emerging from the ten studies they reviewed, clearly suggests that flaxseeds have the potential to decrease breast cancer risk. The study also found that among women living with breast cancer, those who consumed flaxseeds often, were found to live longer.[29]

In 2013 another Canadian study was published in the journal *Cancer Causes & Control*. The study used a food frequency questionnaire to measure the consumption of flaxseed and flax bread by 2,999 women with breast cancer and 3,370 healthy control women who participated in the Ontario Women's Diet and Health Study. It also found that the consumption of flaxseed and flax bread was associated with a reduced breast cancer risk.[30] Other studies report that flaxseeds have the ability to reduce metastasis.[31]

It is recommended that ground flaxseeds are used rather than whole, as it is easier for the body to absorb the beneficial omega-3 fatty acids from the ground seeds. Whole flaxseeds usually pass through the intestines undigested, which means that the body does not get all of the benefits from those seeds. Whole seeds can be ground in a coffee grinder. It is best to grind them at the time when they will be consumed, or you may keep them in the refrigerator for one week or approximately ten days in an airtight glass container. Due to their high fatty acid content, they tend to get rancid very easily.

Suggestion:
- Use grated flaxseeds in your muesli, salads, yogurt, and other recipes, as grinding enables the absorption of the beneficial omega-3 fatty acids.

THE OLIVE TREE AS A SYMBOL OF HEALTH THROUGHOUT TIME

Products derived from the olive tree have been used for their medicinal properties for centuries. In civilizations like the Egyptian and the Greek, the olive tree had and still has a very strong cultural and religious symbolism. Even the emblem of the World Health Organization features the rod of Asclepius over a world map surrounded by olive tree branches, chosen as a symbol of peace and health.

OLIVE OIL AS AN ANTICANCER AGENT

As mentioned earlier, the traditional healthy Mediterranean diet has long been proposed as an ideal dietary model for cancer prevention in Western countries. High consumption of olive oil is the hallmark of the traditional Mediterranean diet.

In the last few decades, the beneficial effects of virgin olive oil have been extensively studied. Virgin olive oil has been found to possess antioxidant, anti-inflammatory, anticancer, antimicrobial, antiviral, anti-atherogenic, and hypoglycemic properties. It is also known for its liver, heart, and brain protecting effects.[32]

Both olives and olive oil contain substantial amounts of various compounds that are considered to be active anticancer agents.[33] The monounsaturated fatty acids of olive oil and its abundant antioxidant components are responsible for these beneficial effects.[34]

The high content of oleic acid in olive oil makes it far less susceptible to oxidation and more stable at high temperatures, compared to other vegetable oils, such as peanut, palm, soybean, and sunflower oils, which are rich in omega-6 fatty acids.

EXTRA VIRGIN OLIVE OIL

We should emphasize the extra benefits and superior quality of extra-virgin olive oil. It is the best type of olive oil, made with the most natural way: simply by crushing olives and extracting the juice. Other olive oils are extracted using chemicals and are even diluted with cheaper oils.

Extra virgin olive oil is rich in phenolic antioxidants, including simple phenols, flavonoids, and lignans, which give olive oil the capacity to neutralize free radicals and protect cells from oxidative stress, potentially inhibiting cancer development.[35]

From analysis of different types of olive oil we know that the most active polyphenol, known as oleuropein, is completely absent from plain olive oil, whereas in extra virgin olive oil it is found in significant amounts.[36]

In the traditional Mediterranean diet olive oil consumption is estimated to be around four tablespoons per day. However, an intake of two to three tablespoons per day, according to a person's activity level and energy needs, is adequate to bring about the noted beneficial effects.

THE SECRET OF BITTER OLIVES AND OLIVE TREE LEAVES

Oleuropein, being the most prevalent phenolic component of the olive tree products, has been studied extensively in the last few years for its pharmacological properties. It is the molecule responsible for unprocessed olives' characteristic bitter taste. It is found in large amounts in olive leaves, in the unprocessed olive fruit, and in extra-virgin olive oil. It is also found in small amounts in table olives, but it is completely absent from plain olive oil.

Oleuropein has been referred to as a new class of anticancer compound by many cancer researchers, as it targets multiple steps in cancer progression. As an antioxidant, it may protect cells from genetic damage leading to cancer development, as an anti-angiogenic agent it can prevent tumor progression, and finally, by directly inhibiting cancer cells it can lead to tumor regression.

OLIVE LEAF EXTRACT

As the olive leaf has by far the highest content of this powerful anticancer compound, it is now believed that it might be effective in treating some tumors and cancers, including liver, prostate, colon, skin, and breast cancer. Its anticancer capacity has been shown in a number of lab and animal studies.

As with other natural agents that target multiple pathways, oleuropein treatment in the form of olive leaf extracts could be useful for both the prevention and treatment of cancer together with other therapeutic approaches.[37]

Olive leaf extract is available in the form of capsules or tablets. The higher the concentration of oleuropein in the capsule or tablet, the more effective it's believed to be.

It's always wise to consult with your own natural health practitioner before taking any supplements. Note that olive leaf extract should not be taken if a person is already taking antibiotics, statin drugs, diabetic drugs, or any fungus or mold medicines.

Suggestion:

- Make extra-virgin olive oil the main oil you use in your salads and meals.
- Use at least 3-4 tablespoons per day.

CHAPTER 14

Why You Need a Brazil Nut a Day

IN THE NUTRITION WORLD BRAZIL NUTS are synonymous to the mineral selenium, an essential micronutrient that is vital for the body, as it boosts the immune system, is involved in the antioxidant protection of the body, has a key role in fertility, and helps defend against cancer.

SELENIUM AND HEALTH

Selenium is vital for human health, well-being, and reproduction.

It plays a major role in supporting a healthy immune system and acts as a powerful antioxidant. It helps recycle vitamin C in the body, leading to an improvement in the overall protection of all cells.

Selenium is an important component of antioxidant enzymes. One of these enzymes is glutathione peroxidase, which is considered to be the body's master antioxidant. Glutathione peroxidase has been found to inhibit cancer in high-risk inflammatory conditions such as inflammatory bowel disease and to help the liver detoxify harmful substances.[1,2]

Selenium also helps in the regulation of the metabolism. It enables proper thyroid function, as it is necessary for the production of the thyroid hormones.[3]

SELENIUM AS AN ANTICARCINOGENIC MICRONUTRIENT

Selenium is one of the most important and most studied minerals when it comes to cancer prevention. There is a strong correlation between levels of selenium in the blood and a reduced risk of several types of cancer.[4,5]

Foods high in selenium can help in cancer prevention. Supplements should be avoided, however, as high levels of selenium in the blood have serious toxic effects. Research has shown that there is a very fine line between the amount of selenium that is beneficial and the amount that is harmful. Oral selenium supplements should be considered only when blood levels of selenium are found to be below 120 µg/l. The ideal range for blood selenium levels in adults is between 130 and 150 µg/l.[6]

SELENIUM-RICH FOODS

Selenium is found naturally in the soil and water, from which it eventually makes its way into plants and animals and ultimately into our food chain. Whether a diet can be adequate in selenium depends largely on the selenium content of the soil of each specific area.

Selenium can be found in many everyday foods. The best sources include Brazil nuts, tuna, sunflower and pumpkin seeds, seafood, and whole grains.

In a study published in the *American Journal of Clinical Nutrition* in 2008, it was found that two Brazil nuts per day were as effective in increasing selenium levels and enhancing antioxidant activity as a supplement containing 100 micrograms of selenium per day. The researchers also noted that just one Brazil nut per day would have been enough to raise selenium intake to within recommended intake levels.[7]

Meat, including chicken, turkey, beef, lamb, or pork, can also be a good source of selenium. One can also get selenium from eggs and milk.

Other vegetable sources include button and shitake mushrooms, onions, spinach, garlic, broccoli, and Brussels sprouts.

Suggestions:

- To make sure you are getting the amount of selenium your body needs, simply eat one or two Brazil nuts daily.
- You can eat them on their own or chop and add them in your muesli, yogurt, salad, or rice, or as a topping for your cooked leafy vegetables.

CHAPTER 15

The Benefits of Dark Chocolate: No More Guilt for Loving Your Chocolate

CHOCOLATES ARE INCREASINGLY BEING SEEN as capable of promoting good health, as they are rich sources of protein, magnesium, calcium, iron and other vital nutrients. Dark chocolate is beneficial to the cardiovascular system, may improve brain function and even help in reducing cancer risk.

DARK CHOCOLATE'S HEALTH BENEFITS

What do blueberries, black tea, dark chocolate, and parsley all have in common? They all contain high amounts of flavonoids, a group of phytonutrients well studied for their capacity to promote health and fight cancer.[1]

Dark chocolate is characterized by a high concentration of cocoa and has very little or no milk added. Cocoa, the dried and fermented seeds of the tropical tree *Theobroma cacao*, has the highest flavanol content of all foods on a per-weight basis. Cocoa is particularly rich in a subclass of flavonoids, the flavan-3-ols (epicatechins, catechins, and procyanidins).

For many people cocoa products such as dark chocolate contribute significantly to their total intake of flavonoids. In many countries they constitute a larger proportion of the diet than foods and drinks containing bioactive compounds with similar properties such as green tea.[2]

Epidemiological studies have shown the health-protective effects of cocoa. People of the Kuna tribe living in the San Blas district of Panama, drink a flavanol-rich cocoa as their main beverage. It is estimated that they have one of the most flavonoid-rich diets in the world, and the rate of heart disease and cancer among the Kuna people is significantly lower than that in mainland Panama.[3]

Dark chocolate has recently been discovered to have a number of health benefits, including protection against heart disease, stroke prevention, reduction of hypertension (high blood pressure), regulation of blood sugar, and reduction in risk of type II diabetes.[4]

Dark chocolate also has a powerful antioxidant activity in the body and has been associated with a reduced risk of cancer, especially colon and breast cancer.[5,6,7]

Cocoa also has a positive effect on brain chemistry and physiology and has been used as a mood enhancer for centuries. Indeed, dark chocolate has been proven to increase blood flow to the brain and to the heart. Medical studies also have confirmed that it contains several chemical compounds that have a positive effect on mood and cognitive health.

ADD COCOA POWDER OR DARK CHOCOLATE TO YOUR DIET

Given the strong relationship between mood and the immune system and the potential anticarcinogenic effect of dark chocolate, adding a small amount of dark chocolate to a healthy balanced diet is a wise thing to do.

Even though there has been some controversy in the past, recent studies show that milk does not affect the bioavailability of cocoa powder flavonoids. This is a very important finding, especially for children. In many countries a large number of children and teenagers do not eat enough fruit and vegetables and the main source of flavonoids in their diet is cocoa powder (up to 50 percent of daily total flavonoid intake).[8]

Suggestions:

- Enjoy dark chocolate as a snack two to three times a week. A good portion is around 20 grams, which gives you around 115 calories. If consumed in moderation it can be enjoyed as a healthy snack without affecting your body weight.
- Melt your dark chocolate in a bain-marie and pour over fruits such as strawberries, pineapple, bananas, or raisins or over chopped nuts.
- You could also grate some dark chocolate over your porridge or cooked oats or simply enjoy a cocoa drink a couple of times per week.

CHAPTER 16

Dietary Fiber:
Why We Need More

MOUNTING RESEARCH SUGGESTS that a high-fiber diet can help reduce your risk of premature death from any cause. This was the conclusion published in early 2015 by a team of researchers from the Shanghai Jiaotong University School of Medicine who evaluated results from seventeen different studies tracking nearly one million Europeans and Americans. The protective effects of fiber are related to the fact that it helps to reduce the risk of a number of chronic diseases, including type II diabetes, heart disease, stroke, and cancer.[1]

DIETARY FIBER HELPS PREVENT COLON CANCER

Cancers of the colon and rectum are among the most frequently diagnosed globally. In a campaign of the American Institute for Cancer Research in 2014, it was estimated that up to 50 percent of colorectal cancer cases could be prevented with changes in the diet and lifestyle. Increasing dietary fiber is one of the main dietary changes related to this reduced risk.

A higher fiber intake, achieved through eating more whole grains and high-fiber foods in general (including fruits, vegetables, and beans), is associated with a reduced risk of a variety of types of cancer.[2,3,4,5,6,7,8] In a UK study it was found that for individuals who consumed an average of twenty-four grams of fiber per day, the odds of developing colorectal cancer were 30 percent lower than for individuals who consumed an average of ten grams per day.[9]

FIBER ALSO PROTECTS AGAINST BREAST CANCER

Another significant association between fiber and cancer was reported in 2011 by a group of Chinese researchers. They performed a meta-analysis of ten large prospective studies examining the association between dietary fiber intake and risk of breast cancer in a total of 712,195 participants. They found that a higher intake of dietary fiber was associated with a significantly lower risk of breast cancer. For every 10 grams of dietary fiber added to the diet per day there was a decrease in risk of breast cancer of 7 percent.[10] This protection might be related to dietary fiber's role in decreasing estrogen levels in the blood, in controlling insulin resistance, and in reducing insulin-like growth factors.

TYPES OF FIBER

There are two types of fiber—soluble and insoluble.

Insoluble fibers add bulk to the diet and help prevent constipation. They do not dissolve in water, so they pass through the gastrointestinal tract relatively intact. Insoluble fibers speed up the passage of food and waste through your gut, therefore reducing your exposure to toxic and carcinogenic factors.

Insoluble fibers are mainly found in whole grains, such as whole-wheat products and flours, wheat bran, seeds, nuts, barley, couscous, brown rice, and bulgur and in the seeds and skins of fruit and vegetables.

Soluble fibers such as those found in legumes and oats, are fermented by bacteria in the colon and become short-chain fatty acids, which protect the cells of the large intestine. They also absorb water and form a gel, which slows down digestion. Soluble fibers delay the emptying of your stomach and make you feel full, which helps control weight. Slower stomach emptying also helps in achieving more stable blood sugar levels and improves insulin sensitivity.

Soluble fibers are also found in apples, oranges, pears, strawberries, nuts, flaxseeds, beans, dried peas, blueberries, psyllium, cucumbers, celery, and carrots.

According to studies, it appears that a higher intake of legumes reduces risk of cancer of various types such as stomach, colon-rectum, prostate, and lung cancer.

Even though fiber undoubtedly contributes to overall good health and longevity, the majority of people do not meet the recommended fiber intake guidelines. Increasing fiber intake is a necessary step to ensure maximum protection against cancer.

Suggestions:

- Choose a whole, plant-based diet.
- Eat legumes (such as beans, chickpeas, peas, and lentils) two to three times per week.
- Make vegetables the largest part of your meals and aim to have a couple of vegetarian meals each week.
- Have two to three fruits per day, preferably spread throughout the day.
- If you eat bread and grains, make sure they are whole-grain.

CHAPTER 17

The Anticancer Role of the Microbes within Us

SYMBIOSIS WITH THE MICROBES WITHIN US

Our body is host to about one hundred trillion microorganisms; in fact, the human body contains over ten times more microorganisms than human cells.[1] Our digestive tract is host to more than one thousand different types of bacteria. These bacteria live in our digestive tracts, helping us break down food and absorb nutrients.

All of these bacteria compete for a place in our digestive tracts. Not all bacteria, however, are beneficial and health promoting. Some bacteria are pathogenic and toxin producing. They thrive when people depend on diets that are high in sugar, white flour, and processed foods. An overgrowth of bad bacteria leads to inflammation and chronic illness. Furthermore, the use of antibiotics kills off all good bacteria, leaving the intestinal tract susceptible to an uncontrolled colonization by bad bacteria.

The balance between the beneficial and harmful bacteria determines the health of our digestive system.

SEVENTY TO EIGHTY PERCENT OF OUR IMMUNE SYSTEM LIES IN THE DIGESTIVE TRACT

Even though oncologists and other doctors often neglect this fact, 70 to 80 percent of our immune system is located within the digestive tract. The strong presence of immune cells in the digestive tract is necessary so that we can kill and remove foreign invaders and toxins that come into the body through the food we eat.

THE THERAPEUTIC VALUE OF PROBIOTICS

The therapeutic value of probiotics is often considered to be modern science, but it is actually quite old. The original hypothesis of the positive role played by certain bacteria was first introduced by Russian scientist Élie Metchnikoff. He was a professor at the Pasteur Institute in Paris, and his work on the immune system won him a Nobel prize in 1908.[2] The existence and importance of the microorganisms that share our body space was not generally recognized until the late 1990s. Today it is widely accepted that these microorganisms have a potentially overwhelming impact on human health.

PROBIOTICS: HEALTHY BACTERIA

By ensuring a regular intake of friendly, health-boosting bacteria, we can achieve a balanced intestinal flora. Extensive research on the field of probiotics highlights the importance of a balanced intestinal flora in maintaining a healthy immune system, in the treatment of autoimmune diseases, in reducing allergies and intolerances, and lastly in preventing cancer.

Quoting a definition given by the World Health Organization, probiotics are "live microorganisms which, when administered in an adequate amount, confer a beneficial heath effect to the host".[3] The term "probiotic" is derived from the Greek word "pro," indicating "promote," and "biotic," representing "life."

ANTICANCER MECHANISMS OF PROBIOTICS

Certain probiotics have been reported to activate specific anticancer mechanisms. Mounting evidence suggests that probiotic bacteria improve the internal conditions of the gut by improving the health and growth of the cells that form the lining of the intestines. They reduce DNA damage in intestinal cells and reduce oxidative stress by producing antioxidants.[4]

Probiotics have also been found to detoxify toxic and carcinogenic compounds in the gut such as aflatoxins and to improve the immune response. From lab and animal studies it is also known that probiotics can inhibit cancer progression and produce anticancer compounds that directly kill cancer cells.[5]

Long-term intake of probiotics from yogurt is related to a reduced incidence of colorectal, breast, and bladder cancer.[6]

PROBIOTICS TAKEN TOGETHER WITH CHEMOTHERAPY

In recent studies, lactic acid bacteria enhanced the effectiveness of some common chemotherapy drugs, such as the 5-fluorouracil (5-FU), in patients with colorectal cancer.[7] In other studies, probiotic supplementation reduced the undesirable side-effects of chemotherapy, such as severe diarrhea and abdominal discomfort. Patients receiving probiotic supplementation had fewer infections, needed less hospital care, and required fewer chemotherapy doses as compared to those who did not receive the probiotics.[8]

Caution: People undergoing some types of cancer therapies become immunocompromised. This is mostly the case for people who have been diagnosed with leukemia. In these cases the use of probiotics poses a serious risk of infection and should therefore be avoided.

The health potential of probiotics is enormous, so this is a good time to consider your probiotic intake and to figure out ways of achieving a good probiotic intake.

Suggestions:

- Take probiotics daily.
- To achieve a good probiotic intake through your diet, add a daily portion of kefir or plain sheep's yogurt that contains only milk and lactic acid bacteria.
- Fermented vegetables are another excellent way to supply beneficial bacteria. Sauerkraut, pickles, and kimchi are good examples of fermented vegetables. Sauerkraut or "sour cabbage" originates from Germany and is made up of finely cut cabbage that has been fermented by lactic acid bacteria. Kimchi is a traditional fermented Korean main dish made of vegetables with a variety of seasonings.
- Miso, natto, and tempeh are fermented traditional products from soy. They originate from Asiatic cuisine and they can contribute to our intake of beneficial probiotic bacteria.
- Introduce your probiotics gradually, beginning with a small dose (i.e., one teaspoon of sauerkraut or kimchi with a meal) and increasing your dose gradually, as tolerated.

CHAPTER 18

Tips on Cooking Methods and Food Combinations for Maximum Protection

COOKING: HOW TO BEST PRESERVE THE ANTICANCER PROPERTIES OF FOODS

In the previous chapters we have explored the foods that promote anticancer activity within the body. By now I am sure you've created a new shopping list in your mind and plan to get started with new recipes and new meals.

Yet how does cooking affect the bioactive compounds in each of the anticancer foods in your list? How does cooking affect their absorption by the body and their ability to defend us against cancer, kill cancer cells, prevent them from spreading, and if necessary help the body recover?

When it comes to cancer protection, it's not only what you eat but also how you cook and prepare your food that is important! In 2013 the American Institute for Cancer Research published a set of practical cooking tips to help people get the most out of their healthy meals.[1]

BROCCOLI

Steaming for up to five minutes is the best way to preserve the enzyme myrosinase, which is found in broccoli and is essential for the formation of the cancer-fighting substance sulforaphane. Steaming the broccoli for more than five minutes, microwaving, or any other method of cooking, such as boiling or cooking it in the oven, destroys this enzyme and damages the anticancer properties of this vegetable.

TOMATOES

Cook tomatoes for a few minutes to release lycopene and to make it more easily absorbed. Add a little olive oil to cooked tomatoes to further enhance the absorption of lycopene. This method of cooking significantly increases the antioxidant and anticancer capacity of tomatoes as compared to eating them raw.

GARLIC

The best way to bring out the health-promoting benefits of garlic is to mince, slice, press, or chop it and then wait for ten to fifteen minutes before cooking it. This delay allows an enzyme found in garlic to mix and react with garlic components and produce allicin. Allicin is the active phytonutrient that has been linked to cancer prevention. Heating destroys the enzyme capable for the formation of allicin.

ADD SOME HEALTHY FATS TO ABSORB FAT-SOLUBLE VITAMINS

The body needs a helping hand from fat to absorb fat-soluble vitamins. Beta-carotene and vitamins A, E, and K are better absorbed when you serve or cook your vegetables with some healthy fats. So serve or cook your green, red, orange, and yellow vegetables with olive oil and add a few nuts or an avocado for more flavor and better health.

FRUITS AND VEGETABLES

The skin of fruits and vegetables is packed with cancer-fighting phytonutrientss. The colorful skins are much denser with protective compounds than the flesh of the fruits and vegetables, and some of these compounds are found only in the skin. For example, eating an apple with its skin on gives you 75 percent more quercetin, the major cancer-fighting phytonutrient, than eating a peeled apple.

Exposing vegetables to high temperatures and cooking them in water significantly reduces the amount of water-soluble vitamins such as vitamin C and folic acid. It is much better to eat your vegetables raw, or if you want them cooked simply steam them, bake them in the oven at a low temperature, or stir-fry them lightly.

SYNERGISTIC EFFECTS OF PROTECTIVE FOODS

In order to explore the protective effects of the foods we eat on health, scientists have been isolating and studying vitamins, nutrients, and other naturally occurring compounds from various foods.

In recent years it has become apparent that foods and food ingredients do not act in isolation, but rather in synergy with one another. Food synergy is defined as the additive or more than additive influence of dietary patterns, foods, and food constituents on health.[2]

There are many examples of nutritional synergism. Nutrient, food, or food and drug combinations augment each other to achieve greater healing capacity. This means that in some cases lower doses are required when nutrients or foods are used synergistically.

We can benefit from the current scientific knowledge of the synergistic effects of protective foods in order to optimize and multiply the preventative and healing value of our diet.

TOMATO PRODUCTS VERSUS LYCOPENE

The majority of studies looking at the protective effects of tomatoes focus on lycopene. Lycopene is the carotenoid in tomatoes that has the strongest antioxidant capacity. In an animal study, lycopene intake was not effective in changing the progression of carcinogenesis, whereas a tomato powder significantly inhibited the progression of prostate cancer. This study suggests that tomato products contain a variety of anticancer compounds in addition to lycopene that act in synergy to affect prostate carcinogenesis.[3]

TOMATO AND BROCCOLI

In a study published in the medical journal *Cancer Research* in 2007, when tomato and broccoli were given together they were more effective at slowing tumor growth than either tomato or broccoli alone.[4] The synergy of the two vegetables is an example of the importance of increasing intake of a variety of protective foods.

GREEN TEA AND THERAPEUTIC MUSHROOMS

The anticancer effect of protective mushrooms can be significantly increased by green tea. In a number of studies, mushrooms and green tea have been found to act synergistically in inhibiting the growth and invasive behavior of highly metastatic breast cancer cells.[5,6]

HIGH-DOSE DIETARY ANTIOXIDANTS ENHANCE THE THERAPEUTIC EFFECT OF STANDARD ANTICANCER TREATMENTS

High doses of dietary antioxidants (including vitamin C at the level of 6 to 8 grams) enhance the level of damage to cancer cells achieved by chemotherapy. The antioxidants protect healthy cells from damage and usually are added to the diet a few days before the start of chemotherapy and continue every day until one month after the completion of the therapy. They reduce treatment side effects and therefore allow patients to have more cycles of therapy. Antioxidant therapy acts in synergy with the standard anticancer treatments and has been found to increase the overall survival rate in lung and other cancer patients.[7,8]

SYNERGISTIC EFFECTS OF PHYTONUTRIENTS FROM FRUIT AND VEGETABLES

Thousands of phytonutrients are present in fruits and vegetables. These phytonutrients have an additive and synergistic effect with one another, resulting in strong antioxidant and anticancer activities within the body. No single antioxidant can replace the combination of natural phytonutrients in fruits and vegetables in achieving the desired anticancer and other health benefits.[9]

Different fruits and vegetables have different phytonutrient profiles with different mechanisms for their protective effects, so when they are combined a much stronger protective effect is achieved.

Studies have shown, for example, that the combination of orange, apple, grape, and blueberry displayed a significant synergistic effect in antioxidant activity. When the four fruits were combined, a much lower dose (five times lower) of each fruit was needed in order to achieve the same antioxidant activity as with any one of them alone. The four fruits acted in a synergistic way, pointing to the need to include in our diet a large variety of fruits and vegetables for optimal benefits.

NATURAL PLANT COMPOUNDS IMPROVE EFFICACY OF CHEMOTHERAPY AND RADIATION

Natural compounds can have additive or even synergistic effects when combined with chemotherapy and radiation. They improve the effectiveness of chemotherapy, decrease resistance to chemotherapeutic drugs, protect the body from the negative side effects of cancer treatments, and detoxify the body from toxic chemotherapy drugs.[10]

Catechins from green tea work synergistically with chemotherapy. They have been found to increase the therapeutic effect of chemotherapy treatments in drug-resistant tumors in animal studies.[11] Green tea was able to increase the concentration of chemotherapeutic agents such as doxorubicin in cancer cells but not in healthy cells, enhancing the anticancer activity of the treatment.

Curcumin from the Indian spice turmeric found in curry powder also works in synergy with the traditional cancer treatments. Like the catechins from green tea, curcumin can sensitize many human cancers to chemotherapy and radiation, even cancers that were considered to be resistant to therapy.[12] The use of a curcumin-based, anticancer therapeutic strategy will hopefully allow the use of lower doses of chemotherapeutic drugs and radiation in the future while achieving much better anticancer results.

The concept that cooking methods and food combinations are important when it comes to cancer prevention might be new to you, but following the tips above will make a huge impact in your body's ability to fight cancer and stay healthy.

CHAPTER 19

The Power to Change The Expression of Our Genes: The New Science of Epigenetics

EPIGENETICS EXPLAIN HOW OUR LIFESTYLE CAN SWITCH OUR GENES "ON" AND "OFF"

The advancement of genetic science in the last fifteen years has led to great discoveries that have opened a completely new road for cancer prevention and treatment.

Recent studies provide substantial evidence that our lifestyle can affect the way our genes are expressed, or "tuned." The potential for change in our genes is known as epigenetics. "Nutri-epigenetics" is the term used to describe how nutrition influences our genes.

Epigenetics describes a series of biological processes that switch our genes "on" and "off" by causing blockages around our DNA. These changes can greatly affect the process of cancer formation and progression.[1]

Our environmental exposures during development in the womb and after birth, as well as our lifelong diet and lifestyle, all affect our cancer risk.[2] Accumulation of epigenetic changes as we age could explain the vast majority of cancers.

Professor Martin Widschwendter, at the University College London, indicates through his work that a series of epigenetic changes that occur through our lifetime can switch our genes on and off, leading to increased cancer risk. For example, the risk of cancer in women at various stages in their lives depends on environmental exposures they had from the period of their embryonic development in their mother's womb, on their genetic background, on their exposure to chemicals and hormones, and on dietary factors such as a low-folate diet and alcohol intake. Obesity and inflammation are also two crucial factors affecting one's cancer risk.[3]

CHANGE YOUR DIET TO CHANGE GENE EXPRESSION AND CANCER RISK

Researchers have discovered that the foods we eat and their bioactive compounds have the potential to change the way our genes behave. This interaction between our genes and our diet ultimately changes our risk for cancer and enables us to offer new therapeutic applications of natural compounds against cancer.

Emerging evidence suggests that the protective effect of the natural compounds described in the previous chapters of this book is achieved through epigenetic mechanisms. Some examples of compounds with epigenetic potential in changing cancer risk are the bioactive compounds in broccoli and cauliflower, vitamin E, and dietary fiber.

EPIGENETIC CHANGES DEREGULATE HEALTHY CELLS

During carcinogenesis (the process of cancer initiation and development), major cell functions and pathways become deregulated. This deregulation affects: (a) cells' potential to repair damage in their DNA, (b) cells' response to inflammation, (c) cells' growth, and (d) how cells multiply.

The latest research on cancer genetics now indicates that these cellular defects are due to epigenetic changes. For example, epigenetic changes can "turn on" or "turn off" the body's detoxifying enzymes. Similarly, they can "turn on" and "turn off" tumor suppressor genes and regulate the life cycle of various cells in the body.

SOME BASIC KNOWLEDGE ON GENETICS

- The DNA is responsible for storing and transferring genetic information in living organisms.
- The three main mechanisms involved in the occurrence of epigenetic changes are: (1) changes in DNA methylation, (2) histone modification, and (3) RNA silencing.
- DNA methylation plays an important role for epigenetic gene regulation in development and disease.
- Histones are proteins that package and compact the long DNA chains. Histone modifications act in diverse biological processes such as gene regulation and DNA repair.
- RNA is responsible for carrying out DNA's blueprint guidelines by transferring the genetic code needed for the creation of proteins that will act as enzymes, body tissues, and the like.

PROTECTIVE NUTRI-EPIGENETIC CHANGES

Dr. Alexander Link, at the Gastrointestinal Cancer Research Laboratory of Baylor University Medical Center in Dallas, has identified dietary polyphenols as an epigenetic factor providing a strong cancer-preventing effect.[4] With his research he also proves that epigenetic factors such as diet and the environment can act together with genetic factors to influence the risk of a normal tissue developing into cancer.

A review article published in 2013 in the journal *Nutrition and Cancer* gives an overview of the research on bioactive components and their influence on the major epigenetic mechanisms in cancer.[5] The evidence presented in this review article can be seen as the cornerstone of a new era in which natural compounds found in common foods can be used as a weapon in the fight against cancer.

From this exciting article I present a few examples of important nutrition and gene interactions, such as: (a) the role of folate in protecting the DNA, (b) the ability of green tea to block cancer cell growth, and (c) the ability of curcumin to cause death among pancreatic and breast cancer cells.

A VITAMIN FOUND IN GREEN VEGETABLES PROTECTS THE DNA

Folate, a B vitamin that is found in green, leafy vegetables, is involved in DNA synthesis and DNA methylation. Extensive evidence suggests that folate deficiency plays a significant role in the development of cancer by damaging the DNA.

In their article "Chemoprevention of Colon Cancer by Calcium, Vitamin D and Folate: Molecular Mechanisms," Sergio A. Lamprecht and Martin Lipkin describe how a low folate intake from the diet leads to an increased risk of colon cancer. A low-folate diet results in reduced DNA methylation and faulty DNA synthesis. This further leads to chromosome instability, chromosome breakage, and increased risk of dangerous mutations that lead to colon cancer.[6]

GREEN TEA BLOCKS CANCER CELL GROWTH WITH EPIGENETIC MECHANISMS

Another example of nutri-epigenetics is the effect of green tea on cancer prevention. EGCG, the major active phytonutrient in green tea with strong antioxidant activity, has been shown to inhibit tumor invasion and angiogenesis. In laboratory studies, EGCG decreased the DNA methylation of cancer cells, resulting in the inhibition of their growth, in restoring normal gene expression, and in a reduction in their capacity for metastasis.

A COMPOUND IN CURRY POWDER INHIBITS CANCER GROWTH BY EPIGENETIC MECHANISMS

A last example of the role of nutri-epigenetics is the effect of curcumin on micro RNA expression. Curcumin, the bioactive ingredient in turmeric found in curry powder, is an herb whose anti-inflammatory and other medicinal properties are recently being extensively studied. Curcumin has been shown to change the micro RNA expression profile of human pancreatic and breast cancer cells. In laboratory studies, curcumin led to significant genetic changes (up-regulation of miRNA-22 and down-regulation of miRNA-199a), leading to inhibition of metastasis and tumor growth and eventually to cancer cell death.[7]

EPIGENETICS TODAY AND TOMORROW

There are still many questions to be answered on nutri-epigenetics, such as the optimal duration and the dose necessary for their preventive effects. The knowledge already gained from the study of epigenetics is a great promise for the future in the fight against cancer.

There is at the moment enough knowledge on epigenetics that can be applied to empower our efforts to prevent and treat cancer. Epigenetic modifications are heritable, which means that they can be transferred to the next generations. Having read up to this point the protective effects of foods and their bioactive components in relation to cancer, it is important to acknowledge that most of these effects are mediated through epigenetic mechanisms.

PART E

Avoid the Foods that Promote Cancer

CHAPTER 20

Sugar

CANCER DEPENDS ON SUGAR

Researchers have long suspected that sugar is involved in the causation of cancer.

The discovery that cancer cells have their own very specific metabolism and that they require more sugar than healthy cells do first became known back in the 1920s. Otto Warburg received a Nobel Prize in 1931 for his research on cancer cell physiology, and his discovery actually revealed one of the hallmarks of cancer.[1] Today the increased dependence of cancer cells on sugar is considered by many cancer researchers to be cancer's Achilles' heel.

Cancer survival depends on sugar. You cannot treat cancer while consuming a high-sugar diet. The most recent research has proved that trying to beat cancer while eating a diet that constantly raises blood glucose is like trying to put out a forest fire while throwing gasoline on the trees.

Just a short walk through any supermarket reveals that most of the foods offered are processed and loaded with sugar. High sugar intake is one of the main reasons behind today's worldwide obesity epidemic, and foods that are high in sugar increase the risk of cancer both directly and indirectly.

HIGH BLOOD SUGAR, INSULIN, AND CANCER

Today cancer is considered to be more a metabolic disease than a genetic one.

Parameters of human metabolism, such as the levels of fasting glucose (sugar) in the blood, are related to cancer risk. The higher the blood sugar level, the higher the risk, especially for pancreatic and liver cancers.[2,3]

Eating foods that are high in sugar and white flour results in a quick rise in blood glucose levels. The body immediately responds by releasing insulin into the blood in order to remove the excess glucose from the blood and transport it into the cells to be converted into energy.

Insulin resistance that occurs in people with type II diabetes and pre-diabetes (also known as metabolic syndrome) leads to constant high levels of glucose (sugar) and insulin in the blood, both of which have been shown to promote the growth of cancer cells.[4] People with type II diabetes have an increased risk of developing several types of cancers.

Until recently, the increased risk of cancer due to high levels of blood glucose was just a hypothesis. In January 2014, however, a study published in the *Journal of Clinical Investigation* by Yasuhito Onodera and his team proved for the first time that increased amounts of sugar in the blood activate certain metabolic pathways within normal cells that initiate cancer formation.[5] Results from the same study prove that a significant reduction in the available sugar leads to a reversal of the cancer cells toward their pre-cancer healthy structure and function.

NINE OUT OF TEN PRE-DIABETIC PEOPLE ARE NOT AWARE OF IT

It is very interesting and surprising that very often cancer patients do not know that they have high blood sugar levels. A study published in 2011 in the *Journal of the American Society of Clinical Oncology* followed three thousand women with breast cancer. The study found that 60 percent of the breast cancer patients who had diabetes and 90 percent of those in a pre-diabetic state did not know it.[6]

GROWTH FACTORS RELATED TO INSULIN (IGF-1) STIMULATE CANCER GROWTH

Another important factor in the causation of cancer is a molecule that is released together with insulin, called insulin-like growth factor-1. As its name implies, IGF-1 is a local tissue growth factor that promotes cell growth. High levels of IGF-1 are released with high carbohydrate diets, and these high levels of IGF-1 are associated with increased cancer risk, more rapid cancer growth, and metastasis.

A large analysis of seventeen studies from twelve countries clearly showed that women's IGF-1 levels were related to a higher risk of breast cancer.[7] Other large meta-analyses indicate that high IGF-1 levels are also associated with the risk of colorectal, prostate, and pancreatic cancers.

Research also shows that IGF-1 has anti-apoptotic effects, which means that it prevents cancer cells from dying. This unfortunately leads to a decreased sensitivity to the drugs used for chemotherapy.[8] Insulin and IGF-1 are also involved in cancer formation and progression by promoting inflammation.

A diet that prevents high blood glucose and high levels of insulin and IGF-1 can help to:

1. Prevent cancer formation and development
2. Prevent metastasis
3. Reduce inflammation
4. Improve prognosis and prolong disease-free years of life in cancer patients
5. Improve chemotherapy effectiveness in certain cancers.

SUGAR INTAKE DAMAGES THE DNA OF IMMUNE CELLS

A sugar-loaded fizzy drink per day can damage human immune cells to the same level as cigarette smoking! The team of Dr. Elissa Epel from the University of California San Francisco studied the effect of sugar on the immune system. In a study that they published in December 2014, they found that the length of the telomeres in the DNA of human immune cells is shorter in people who drink sugary fizzy drinks daily. DNA telomeres are something like the plastic end of a shoelace that prevents it from unraveling. Shorter telomeres are linked to an aging immune system, to an increased risk of cancer, and to shorter life spans.[9]

WHAT CAUSES HIGH BLOOD SUGAR?

Foods and snacks that are high in simple sugars and in refined, processed carbohydrates like white flour increase blood glucose and insulin levels sharply after they are eaten. Examples of these foods are pastries, sweets, candies, white bread, most breakfast cereals, juices and soft drinks, white and brown sugar, and honey.

In non-athletes, a diet rich in these kinds of foods leads to long-term metabolic dysfunction, insulin resistance, excess weight and obesity, and over time to increased risk of type II diabetes and cancer.[10]

BODY WEIGHT AND THE EFFECTS OF DIETARY CARBOHYDRATES ON CANCER RISK

The type of carbohydrates eaten is more important for people who are overweight and who do not exercise, probably because of insulin resistance.[11] A study by Dominique S. Michaud at the US National Cancer Institute found that pancreatic cancer risk was increased by a diet rich in carbohydrates only in people who had insulin resistance.[12]

KEEP YOUR SUGAR AND CARBOHYDRATE INTAKE UNDER CONTROL

For the prevention of cancer, one should aim to maintain a healthy weight and to exercise regularly. These are lifestyle steps that will help you maintain good control of blood glucose, avoid insulin resistance, and prevent type II diabetes.

Good blood sugar control can be achieved through reducing the quantity of carbohydrates altogether, such as the refined carbohydrates in most flour products, and avoiding simple carbohydrates. This means avoiding sugar, honey, maple syrup, molasses, products with corn syrup and high-fructose corn syrup, as well as sweetened soft drinks and fruit juices as much as possible.

In order to achieve good glycemic control after meals, the amount of carbohydrate rich foods must be limited. The amount of protein and fat of a meal also influence the blood glucose response. As the amount of proteins and fat increase, meals get digested more slowly and result in better glycemic control. Proteins from fish, chicken, pulses, seeds and seeds and good fats from olive oil, coconut oil and avocado contribute to a good blood sugar control.

SUGAR MAKES CANCER MUCH MORE DEADLY

Research has shown that chronic and untreated high blood sugar increases the risk of life-threatening complications, promotes cancer growth, and reduces survival times in early-stage cancer patients.[13, 14] For this reason, strict control of blood sugar is a key factor for improving prognosis.

One large study on sugar intake in cancer patients was carried out by Dr. Colleen Huber and her colleagues at Nature Works Best Cancer Clinic, a naturopathic cancer clinic in the United States. Their seven-year-long ongoing study involved 317 cancer patients and the results of the study were reported in the *Cancer Strategies Journal*, in the spring of 2014. The clinic recommended that all cancer patients avoid all sweetened foods and drinks. Regardless of the type of cancer or the stage, the study showed that cancer patients who were avoiding sugar had more than twice the survival rate (90 percent) of the sugar eaters (36 percent).[15]

It is very important that people who have cancer keep their blood glucose levels under very tight control. Both fasting glucose levels (a measurement of blood sugar in the morning before having anything to eat) and HbA1c (a long-term indicator of glucose levels) should be measured and monitored frequently.

Keeping an eye on your blood glucose levels and making the right changes in your diet to ensure a good blood sugar control are key elements in cancer prevention and in improving the results of any chosen cancer therapy. Follow the suggestions below to optimize your blood glucose metabolism.

Suggestions:

- Limit the amount of sugar in the diet. Avoid completely simple sugars such as sweetened drinks, sugar in desserts, honey, molasses, juices, and the like.
- Switch to a diet of whole, unprocessed foods. Eat most foods in their unprocessed state (i.e., eat dried beans that you've cooked yourself rather than buying tinned baked beans and choose whole-grain breads, pasta, and wild rice).
- Avoid processed foods with sugar and high-fructose corn syrup such as cookies, cakes, sodas, soft drinks, and other sweets.
- Limit desserts to special occasions.
- Eat natural sugars such as honey, molasses, and maple syrup in very small amounts, as they, too, increase blood sugar levels significantly.
- Eat large amounts of vegetables with all meals.
- If you are overweight, losing weight will help in achieving better blood sugar control. Test your fasting blood sugar levels (morning) and HβA1c (long-term estimation of blood glucose levels) often in order to detect at the earliest stages any metabolic effects leading to type II diabetes. Reduce the overall quantity of your meals and snacks, reduce the carbohydrates you eat, avoid sugar and sugary snacks and increase exercise. If needed your doctor might advise the initiation of medication that helps in reducing blood sugar levels such as metformin. Metformin is related to a reduced cancer risk among people with Type II diabetes.[16, 17]

- Increase the good fats in your diet such as olive oil, nuts, seeds and nut-butters (i.e. peanut butter), avocados and coconut oil. High fat meals delay digestion and stomach emptying, leaving foods in the stomach longer and delaying the absorption of glucose into the blood.
- Prefer to eat your pasta al-dente as overcooking increases the glycemic index of foods.
- If needed add small amounts of stevia in your diet until you manage to gradually let go the need for sweets. You can also use a little stevia in your baking as a sugar substitute.

CHAPTER 21

Caution with Eating Meat

WITH SO MANY DIET MODELS claiming to be the healthiest today, it has become extremely difficult for the average person to decide how much, if any meat should be eaten. These popular diet models range from vegan and vegetarian diets to the paleo diet (a diet model based on the diets of our Paleolithic ancestors which is translated to a high meat diet). Scientists have been evaluating the link between meat consumption and cancer for many years now.

THE WORLD CANCER RESEARCH FUND RECOMMENDS LIMITING RED MEAT CONSUMPTION

In November 2007, the American Institute for Cancer Research (AICR) and the World Cancer Research Fund (WCRF) published a report on the prevention of cancer. This expert report, titled, *"Food, Nutrition, Physical Activity and the Prevention of Cancer: A Global Perspective,"* is still considered to be the most comprehensive report on diet and cancer ever completed.[1]

The expert panel of world-renowned scientists in the field developed ten recommendations for cancer prevention, one of which is to limit consumption of red meats and avoid processed meats. The expert panel that reviewed all of the relevant scientific studies concluded that there is convincing evidence that red meat consumption is a cause of colorectal cancer. The American Institute for Cancer Research has assigned red meat to Group 2A as being a probable carcinogen to humans.

Red meat contains substances that are especially linked to colon cancer. Studies also show that people who eat a lot of red meat usually eat fewer plant-based foods that are rich in cancer-protective properties.

WHAT DO WE MEAN BY RED MEAT?

Red meat refers to beef, pork, lamb, and goat and includes foods like hamburgers, steak, pork chops, and roast lamb. The WCRF report emphasizes that it does not recommend a meat-free diet or a diet containing no foods of animal origin, as it considers that many foods of animal origin are nourishing and healthy if consumed in modest amounts.

WHAT IS THE GOAL FOR WEEKLY CONSUMPTION?

The American Institute for Cancer Research recommends limiting the weekly consumption of red meat to 500 grams (18 ounces) of cooked red meat per week. This goal corresponds to the level of consumption of red meat above which the risk of colorectal cancer can clearly be seen to rise. Based on the results of all the relevant research studies on the role of red meat and cancer, we recommend an even lower amount of red meat, of approximately 300 grams per week.

As a rough guide to meat portion sizes, one deck of cards or the inside of an average person's palm is approximately 85 to 100 grams of cooked meat.

HOW RED MEAT INCREASES CANCER RISK

Red meat can increase cancer risk in a number of ways. The heme iron of red meat has been found to cause damage to the internal wall (lining) of the colon. Iron itself has been linked to an increased production of free radicals, which can lead to DNA damage, inflammation, and other toxic effects to the cells, further leading to the initiation and progression of colon carcinogenesis.[2]

The cooking method used for preparing red meat, the type and quality of the animals' feed, and the exposure of the animals to growth hormones, pesticides, or antibiotics all play a role in determining whether the meat we eat affects our risk for developing cancer.

RECENT STUDIES CONFIRM THE RECOMMENDATIONS FOR LOWERING CONSUMPTION OF RED MEAT

Large studies published after the WCRF and AICR report support and confirm the association between red meat and cancer. One of these studies is the Nurses' Health Study, which followed 83,767 participants for around thirty years.[3] Among the participants of this large study, women who consumed one serving of red or processed meat daily had a 20 percent increased risk of colon cancer as compared with women who did not eat any red or processed meat.

Another study published shortly after the WCRF and AICR recommendations reported the findings of the US National Institutes of Health (NIH) Diet and Health Study. This study investigated whether red or processed meat intake increases cancer risk at a variety of sites by following approximately five hundred thousand people for around eight years. The researchers found significantly elevated risks (ranging from 20 percent to 60 percent) for esophageal, colorectal, liver, and lung cancer among the people who had the highest red meat intake when compared to those with the lowest intake. Furthermore, individuals in the highest quintile of processed meat intake had a 20 percent elevated risk for colorectal and a 16 percent elevated risk for lung cancer.[4]

From the NIH study it can be estimated that if people were reducing their red meat intakes to the levels of the group with the lowest intake, 33 percent of esophageal, 9 percent of colorectal, 35 percent of liver, and 10 percent of lung cancer cases could be prevented.

WHAT ABOUT PROCESSED MEAT?

The term "processed" refers to meats preserved by smoking, curing, or salting, or by the addition of chemical preservatives. Examples include ham, bacon, pastrami, salami, and pepperoni, as well as hot dogs, sausages, corned beef, pate, tinned meat, and deli/luncheon meats.

The review of the research by WCRF and the AICR concluded that eating processed meat is linked to increased risk of cancer and particularly of colorectal cancer. Unlike red meat, however, no safe level of intake exists, as even a low intake of processed meat increases cancer risk. Results from the European Prospective Investigation into Cancer and Nutrition (EPIC) Study published in 2013 found significantly higher all-cause mortality with higher consumption of processed meat.[5]

On October 26, 2015, the International Agency for Research on Cancer (IARC) classified processed meat as a carcinogen. To reach this conclusion, twenty-two experts from ten countries reviewed more than eight hundred studies and found that eating fifty grams of processed meat every day increased the risk of colorectal cancer by 18 percent. That's the equivalent of about four strips of bacon or one hot dog.[6]

Nitrites and nitrates are the most commonly used preservatives. They are added in order to preserve the color and extend the shelf life of processed meats by preventing contamination with pathogenic bacteria. They may be related to the increased cancer risk observed, as together with the protein of meat they form cancer-causing nitrosamines. Some processed meats may also increase cancer risk as a result of the smoking process to which they are exposed, which leads to the formation of cancer-causing polycyclic aromatic hydrocarbons. High amounts of salt also used as a method for preserving meat can promote the development of stomach cancer.

AVOID SMOKE AND HIGH TEMPERATURES WHEN COOKING MEAT

When meat is cooked at high temperatures (i.e., when grilling, barbequing, or frying), two major cancer promoters are produced. These compounds, known as heterocyclic amines and polycyclic aromatic hydrocarbons (PAH), can damage DNA and lead to an increased risk of cancer.

To avoid the formation of these carcinogenic compounds it is best to cook your meat at lower temperatures and to avoid direct exposure of meat to an open flame.

Polycyclic aromatic hydrocarbons are formed when fat drips onto the heat source (i.e., the coals), causing excess fumes and smoke. The smoke surrounds the food, transferring cancer-causing PAHs to the meat. To reduce the amount of PAH, avoid cooking fatty meats and trim off the visible fat before you grill.

Heterocyclic amines are formed when meat is cooked at high temperatures and especially when meat is well done or slightly burnt. Several studies have found a link between high intakes of well-done, fried, or barbequed meat and colorectal, pancreatic, and breast cancer and between cooked meat in general and stomach cancer.[7] People eating medium-well or well-done beef, for example, were more than three times more likely to develop stomach cancer as compared to those who ate rare or medium-rare beef.

COOKING TIPS FOR RED MEAT

Avoiding overcooked meat can make a big difference in the cancer risk to which it exposes you. Never eat charred or burned meat (the brown or black parts). Well-done and char-grilled meats that are slightly burnt on the outside are among the worst foods in increasing the risk of cancer. Another way to reduce heterocyclic amines is to flip your meat often to minimize the chance of it getting burned.

Keeping meat moist while cooking generates fewer heterocyclic amines, so prefer stewing, boiling, steaming, or poaching and generally cooking methods that are liquid based.

Marinating meat can significantly reduce the production of heterocyclic amines. By marinating meat in olive oil or vinegar you can prevent the formation of these carcinogenic compounds by 90 percent. Mixing the marinade together with herbs and spices further enhances its protective effect.

Researchers have also tested marinating steaks in beer or red wine for four to six hours before grilling them to well done on a charcoal grill. Interestingly, these alcoholic marinades were able to reduce carcinogenic compounds by 60 to 90 percent. Black beer marinade (made from a dark lager) and red wine marinade had the most protective effect.

HOW ARE THE ANIMALS FED AND RAISED?

When considering your red meat options, it is worth pointing that not all red meat is the same. The quality and health benefits of meat can be affected greatly by the type of feed the animal receives and how it is raised.

Grass-fed beef is higher in omega-3 fatty acids and contributes to a better omega-6 to omega-3 ratio. It also has a higher level of conjugated linolenic acid, CLA, a group of fatty acids that inhibit carcinogenesis. Grass-fed beef is higher in precursors for Vitamin A and E and higher in cancer-fighting antioxidants as compared to grain-fed beef. Grass-fed beef also tends to be lower in overall fat content and is generally considered to be of much better nutritional quality.[8]

Organically grown red meat is also much cleaner. Conventional meat is very often raised with significant amounts of hormones and antibiotics and fed with pesticide-originating feeds.

A Spanish study published in 2014 found that conventional meat and meat products were the main dietary factors contributing to human contamination with environmental pollutants. Sausage and meat consumption increased the probability of having detectable levels of dioxin-like PCBs in the blood.[9]

Persistent organic pollutants such as PCBs and chlorinated pesticides have well-known toxic and carcinogenic effects. Chronic exposure to these compounds is particularly harmful for the liver and thyroid gland. In addition, chronic exposure to PCBs and chlorinated pesticides is considered to be a risk factor for developing diseases such as obesity, metabolic syndrome, diabetes, and cancer.

WHAT ABOUT WHITE MEAT AND FISH?

For the prevention of cancer, the American Cancer Society specifically advises limiting the intake of red and processed meats and choosing fish and poultry as lean alternatives instead of beef, pork, or lamb.[10]

In a large U.S. study that followed 492,186 participants over a period of nine years, poultry and fish intake was associated with lower risk of digestive and respiratory cancers.[11] This protective effect was largely due to the substitution of red meat with poultry and fish. Simply increasing fish or poultry intake without reducing red meat intake may be less beneficial for cancer prevention.

In comparison to red meat, poultry and fish are lower in saturated fat and heme iron, potential factors leading to oxidative stress and DNA damage when red meat is consumed. Consumption of white meat is also likely to result in significantly lower exposure to carcinogenic nitrosamines, which form more readily with red and processed meat intake.

STILL BE CAREFUL WHEN COOKING WHITE MEAT AND FISH AND WHEN CHOOSING FISH

One must remain careful when choosing fish and when cooking poultry or fish.

High cooking temperatures, exposure to smoke, and over-cooking or burning can lead to the formation of the same carcinogenic compounds in poultry or fish that are formed in red meat. For example, high levels of heterocyclic amines have been found in fried fish and fish cooked at high temperatures, and polycyclic aromatic hydrocarbons are deposited on the surface of smoked or grilled fish.[12,13] Smoked or salted fish have been found to increase the risk of advanced prostate cancer.[14]

Furthermore, some species of fish may be a source of potential carcinogens, such as PCBs, dioxins, and mercury.

As with red meat, keeping white meat and fish moist while cooking generates fewer heterocyclic amines. Stewing, boiling, steaming, or poaching should be preferred. Also, marinating chicken and other white meat or fish in olive oil with the addition of herbs can significantly reduce the production of heterocyclic amines.

VEGETARIAN DIETS HAVE A REDUCED CANCER RISK

In a number of large studies vegetarians have been found to have a lower incidence of all cancers as compared to meat eaters. One of these studies was led by Professor Timothy J Key, a leading UK cancer epidemiologist and director of the Cancer Epidemiology unit at the University of Oxford. Professor Tim Key is the principal investigator of the Oxford cohort of sixty-five thousand British participants taking part in the largest ever European study into cancer and nutrition, known as the EPIC study.

In a recent analysis published in 2014, Professor Key's team reported data gathered from two of the largest prospective studies in the United Kingdom. One was the Oxford Vegetarian Study and the second involved the UK participants in the EPIC study. They found total cancer incidence to be 12 percent lower in fish eaters, 11 percent lower in vegetarians, and 19 percent lower in vegans as compared with meat eaters.[15]

A very important finding from the analysis of these two studies was that incidence of stomach cancer was 63 percent lower among vegetarians and vegans as compared with meat eaters. Also, colorectal cancer risk was 34 percent lower in fish eaters than in meat eaters.

Results from large US studies also show lower cancer risk among vegetarians. For example, in the Adventist Health Study II, total cancer risk was found to be significantly lower in vegetarians and in vegans than in nonvegetarians, by 8 percent and 16 percent, respectively. Vegetarians had a lower risk of cancers of the gastrointestinal tract, such as colorectal cancer.[16,17]

Diets containing only plant proteins are thought to reduce insulin-like growth factor-1, a growth factor that appears to be important in the development of several types of cancer.

Suggestions:
- Aim not to exceed 300 - 500 grams (11 - 18 ounces) of cooked red meat per week.
- Choose high quality red meat such as organic or grass-fed.
- Try to avoid processed meat altogether.
- Choose mostly fish and poultry as lean alternatives instead of beef, pork, or lamb.

- As with red meat, keep white meat and fish moist while cooking in order to minimize the heterocyclic amines produced.
- Prefer stewing, boiling, steaming or poaching when cooking your protein foods.
- Marinate meat, chicken and other white meat or fish in olive oil and herbs to significantly reduce the production of the toxic heterocyclic amines.

CHAPTER 22

Acrylamide

WHEN CARBOHYDRATE-RICH FOODS are cooked at high temperatures, a neurotoxic and potentially carcinogenic chemical, known as acrylamide, is produced. In November 2007 the European research project HEATOX concluded that there is strong evidence linking acrylamide to an increased cancer risk.[1,2]

HEATOX also concluded that home-cooked foods contribute far less to overall acrylamide levels than food that is industrially or restaurant prepared. Frying, baking, and broiling are the worst offenders. Longer cooking times increase acrylamide, so try to keep the duration of cooking as short as possible.

Potato chips and French fries have been found to have the highest amounts of acrylamide. The darker brown the food, the more acrylamide it contains. As with potatoes, overheating bread forms acrylamide, and dark brown toast has higher acrylamide levels as compared to light brown toast.

Acrylamide has been found only in foods cooked at over 120 degrees Celsius, so boiling and steaming are not related to acrylamide formation and are much safer methods of cooking.

When it comes to the best diet for cancer, the benefits of a raw diet are often highlighted. The dangerous by-products of heavily cooked or processed foods are among the reasons why raw or lightly cooked foods are the best choice.

Suggestions:

- The best way to minimize acrylamide exposure at home is to avoid overcooking when baking, frying, grilling, roasting, or toasting carbohydrate-rich foods.
- Keep the duration of cooking as short as possible.
- Avoid potato chips and French fries, as they have been found to have the highest amounts of acrylamide.
- Soaking raw potatoes in water for fifteen to thirty minutes prior to roasting has been shown to reduce acrylamide formation during cooking.
- The darker brown the food, the more acrylamide it contains (for instance, dark brown toast compared to light brown toast). The FDA recommends preparing toast until it has a light brown color and not dark brown. If there are very dark areas, avoid eating them.
- Choose boiling and steaming as your preferred method of cooking.
- Store potatoes in a cool dark place such as a cupboard or pantry as this reduced the amount of acrylamide formed while cooking.

CHAPTER 23

Reduce Cancer Risk by Reducing Dietary Salt

LIMIT SALTY FOODS AND FOODS PROCESSED WITH SALT

Salt intake was first reported as a possible risk factor for stomach cancer in 1959. In some early studies the use of refrigerators for food storage, considered to be an indicator of a reduction in the consumption of salted foods, was related with a reduction in stomach cancer rates.[1]

Today most published epidemiological studies provide evidence that a high intake of salt and salted foods contributes to an increased risk of stomach cancer. The recommendations for cancer prevention by the American Institute for Cancer Research (AICR) and the World Cancer Research Fund (WCRF) advise the public to limit consumption of salty foods and foods processed with salt as a strategy to reduce stomach cancer rates.

Gastric cancer is a major health burden worldwide, as it is the second largest cause of cancer deaths after lung cancer. In a study by Peleteiro et al. published in the *British Journal of Cancer* in

2011, people with the highest intake of salt were approximately twice as likely to develop gastric cancer as compared to those with the lowest intake.[2]

SALT AND STOMACH CANCER RISK

Studies have shown that high salt intake can damage the lining of the stomach, leading to gastritis and inflammation. A high salt concentration in the stomach creates conditions that favor infection by *Helicobacter pylori*. Conditions related to high salt concentrations in the stomach then synergize with *Helicobacter pylori* and lead to progression of gastric cancer. *H. pylori* is one of the most important recognized risk factors for gastric cancer. The growth, survival, and virulence of *H. pylori* are increased as salt concentration in the stomach increases.[3]

CUT DOWN SALT IN YOUR DIET

Most of the salt in our diets comes from processed foods. Even foods that do not taste salty are often high in salt. In most developed countries, 80 percent of salt eaten is added to foods at the manufacturing stage by the food industry, so consumers have no say in the amount of salt they are eating.

This is again one of the reasons why a diet consisting of mainly unprocessed foods is better than a diet depending on ready-made meals or snacks.

The most important foods to avoid are heavily salted, smoked, and pickled foods. These foods are very popular in Japan, which explains the high rates of stomach cancer in that country.

Processed meats are also a major source of salt in the diet, together with canned products like soups and sauces. Other high-salt foods include foods with soy sauce, soup powders, frozen meals, pizza, chips, most common breads, and some breakfast cereals.

It is very important to note that highly salted foods and snacks exert an addictive effect, especially on children. They also increase thirst and are related to increased sugary drink consumption and obesity, all factors further increasing cancer risk by other mechanisms. Frequent consumption of very salty foods suppresses the salt taste receptors and increases even further the demand for highly salted products, at the same time reducing the preference for more natural and plain flavors such as those found in fruits and vegetables.

Adding herbs to a cooked meal can help boost its taste while at the same time reducing the need for added salt both in the cooking phase and at the table.

Cutting down salt in your diet is a key factor in reducing cancer risk. Read the suggestions below to take the necessary steps for a low salt diet.

Suggestions:

- Avoid foods that are heavily salted, smoked, or pickled.
- Avoid canned foods and high-salt foods such as foods with soy sauce, soup powders, frozen meals, pizza, chips, most common breads, and some breakfast cereals.
- Choose a diet consisting of mainly unprocessed foods and avoid ready-made meals or snacks.
- Replace salt in your meals with herbs.

CHAPTER 24

Foods That Cause Inflammation and Their Relationship with Cancer

INFLAMMATION HAS LONG BEEN ASSOCIATED with cancer development. Prolonged inflammation can damage your body's healthy cells and researchers have found that many cancers arise from sites of infection, chronic irritation and inflammation.

Chronic inflammation plays a key role at different stages of cancer development.

CHRONIC INFLAMMATION EXPLAINED

Chronic inflammation appears to both initiate and fuel cancer. While acute inflammation is one of the most powerful weapons of our immune system and absolutely necessary for our survival, chronic inflammation creates an environment that supports cancer initiation and growth.

Acute inflammation is a response of our immune system. The immune system is designed to eliminate enemies such as bacteria and toxins and to help in repairing tissues damaged by injury. Tissue swelling, irritation, redness, and pain accompany inflammation.

Chronic inflammation occurs when the immune system keeps on producing inflammatory chemicals even after an acute threat has been settled or in the absence of a real threat. This mistaken and excessive immune response creates chaos instead of repair and results in a "microenvironment" in the body that causes severe damage and contributes to disease.

Chronic and excess inflammation not only supports cancer development but is also considered to be one of the leading drivers of the most serious diseases we are dealing with today, including heart disease, metabolic syndrome, diabetes, arthritis, and Alzheimer's.[1]

A LINK BETWEEN INFLAMMATION AND CANCER: AN OLD THEORY IS NOW PROVEN

The link between inflammation and cancer was first hypothesized by Rudolf Virchow back in 1863, when he found with his microscope immune cells in cancer samples.[2] Virchow was a great German doctor, widely regarded as one of the greatest and most influential physicians in history.

In the traditional Indian natural medicine Ayurveda, the link between inflammation over long periods of time and cancer was written about as far back as five thousand years ago.

However, it was not until the last decade that the hypothesis of Rudolf Virchow was proven with sound scientific evidence. Nowadays it is generally accepted that chronic inflammation increases cancer risk.[3] A number of studies have proven the link between chronic low-level inflammation and many types of cancer, including lymphoma, prostate, ovarian, pancreatic, colorectal, and lung cancer.[4]

Several studies also suggest that measuring inflammation markers at the time of diagnosis and after treatment can predict the survival time for many cancers.[5] Lower levels of inflammation indicate a better prognosis, meaning that the person is more likely to respond well to treatment and live longer.

Inflammation decreases quality of life, impairs immune function and lowers tolerance of some anticancer therapies.

FACTORS CONTRIBUTING TO CHRONIC INFLAMMATION

There are many factors that lead to chronic inflammation. Prolonged exposure to environmental and dietary carcinogens results in low-grade but continuous inflammation of the gastrointestinal tract and liver that acts on all stages of cancer formation. Other types of chronic inflammation, such as autoimmune diseases and obesity, can also promote cancer development and progression. Autoimmune diseases include Hashimoto's thyroiditis, multiple sclerosis, myasthenia gravis, rheumatoid arthritis, inflammatory bowel disease, and celiac disease.

The worldwide obesity epidemic, which is expanding in an uncontrollable manner, results in low-grade chronic inflammation and is considered to be a silent factor contributing to increases in cancer rates. Even though it is quite small and often undetectable, obesity-induced inflammation acts at all stages of cancer development and progression. Chronically high levels of blood glucose and blood insulin as those associated with pre-diabetes or with uncontrolled diabetes contribute too to chronic inflammation.

Chronic inflammation also results from diets which are high in sugar, unhealthy fats, certain food additives and which contain an excess of omega-6 fatty acids.

THE ROLE OF INFLAMMATION IN CANCER DEVELOPMENT

Inflammation acts at all stages of cancer formation, including initiation, promotion, invasion, and metastasis. It may contribute to cancer initiation by causing mutations (damage to the DNA), DNA instability, and epigenetic modifications. Inflammation can turn healthy cells into pre-cancerous (premalignant cells) and enhance their survival. Inflammation also stimulates the formation of new blood vessels that feed the cancer. It also promotes the formation of a hospitable microenvironment in which pre-cancerous cells can survive and expand. Eventually, inflammation also promotes metastatic spread.[6]

Since inflammation is affected by diet and the environment, Sergei Grivennikov, PhD, assistant professor at the School of Medicine of the University of California, has stated that, "One of the major lessons learned from investigating the relationship between inflammation and cancer is that most cancers are preventable."[7]

ANTI-INFLAMMATORY STRATEGIES

In order to keep inflammation to a minimum, we have to balance the factors that promote inflammation with the factors that block it.

Inflammation is caused by smoking, drinking alcohol, poor dietary habits, domestic and outdoor pollution, sleep deficit, and extreme exercise. High levels of stress and ongoing emotional tension also contribute to increasing inflammation levels. It is therefore of great importance for everyone to be aware of and identify the factors that promote inflammation in their own lives and to take specific measures to address these factors.

FOODS AND INFLAMMATION

What we eat can increase or decrease inflammation. The effect of diet on inflammation has been increasingly recognized in the last few years. In late 2014 the first science-based dietary index of inflammation was presented at the American Institute of Cancer Research (AICR) Annual Research Conference.

This index is a tool developed to predict how an individual's diet links to inflammation and to inflammation-related health risks. The team came from the University of South Carolina, and as Susan E. Steck, associate professor and co-author of the related studies, pointed out, "We are now starting to see that diet influences inflammation and that the inflammatory potential of the diet is associated with colorectal cancer."[8]

Their results showed that diets high in fiber, spices such as turmeric and ginger, healthy fats, fish, nuts, and carotenoids from green, leafy vegetables contribute to an anti-inflammatory effect that results in a reduced risk of colorectal cancer.

The index they developed includes foods that have proven links with C-reactive protein (CRP) and other markers of inflammation. An analysis from the Iowa Women's Health Study found that women who consumed the most pro-inflammatory diets were at 20 percent greater risk of colorectal cancer than women with more anti-inflammatory diets.[9]

The findings of the South Californian team concluded that the Western diet that is high in sugar, fried foods, high-fat dairy products, and refined grains is associated with the higher levels of inflammatory biomarkers such as CRP and Interleukin-6 (IL-6).[10]

Suggestions:

- Try to have a diet that is low in sugar.
- Avoid trans fats by avoiding processed and fried foods.
- If you are overweight try to avoid further weight gain and do consider losing weight gradually, by making permanent changes in your diet and increasing your activity levels.
- Do check your blood sugar levels regularly and aim to keep them within the normal range.
- If you have diabetes or are in a pre-diabetic state it is very important to monitor and control your blood glucose levels very carefully. Do measure your HbA1c levels at least 3 times per year, aiming for a value of 6% or less.
- Try to be informed about environmental and dietary carcinogens and minimize your exposure to them.
- If you have an autoimmune disease such as Hashimoto's thyroiditis, multiple sclerosis, myasthenia gravis, rheumatoid arthritis, inflammatory bowel disease, and celiac disease you should be following an anti-infammatory diet very strictly.
- An anti-inflammatory diet is high in fiber, spices such as turmeric and ginger, healthy fats, fish, nuts, and carotenoids from green, leafy vegetables and is low in sugar, fried foods, high-fat dairy products, and refined grains.

CHAPTER 25

Unhealthy Fats:
Excess Omega-6

BOTH THE OMEGA-3 AND OMEGA-6 fatty acids in our diet are "essential." By essential we mean that they cannot be synthesized by the body and must be supplied by our diet. When they enter the body they are biologically active and have important roles in various processes including inflammation and forming our cell membranes.

With regard to inflammation, the omega-6 and omega-3 fatty acids have opposite effects. The omega-6's are pro-inflammatory, while the omega-3's have an anti-inflammatory effect; this is why their presence in the diet should be equivalent.

A diet that is high in omega-6 but low in omega-3 fatty acids leads to excess inflammation in the body. A diet that provides balanced amounts of each reduces inflammation end enables the body to work at its best.[1] Humans therefore need to consume similar amounts of omega-6 and omega-3 fats. The relationship between the two is called the "omega-6 to omega-3 ratio," and a ratio of 2:1 or 3:1 is considered ideal.

Traditional diets where people eat a non-industrial diet have a balanced omega-6 to omega-3 ratio of about 4:1 to 1:4.[2]

In the last one hundred years the consumption of vegetable oils rich in omega-6 has increased dramatically. The problem with the typical Western diet is that most people are now eating way too many omega-6's relative to omega-3's. The ratio today is generally found to be between 15:1 and 40:1. This level of consumption of omega-6 fatty acids is much higher than what we are genetically adapted to.

REDUCE THE OMEGA-6 FATTY ACIDS IN YOUR DIET

Omega-6 fatty acids cause inflammation, and unfortunately they are everywhere. They are used in cooking and baking and they're in packaged food, fast food, and restaurant food.

Omega-6 fats are mainly found in vegetable oils, such as soybean oil and corn oil, but they are also found in peanut oil, grape seed oil, cotton seed oil, safflower oil, and sunflower oil.

Butter, coconut oil, palm oil, and olive oil, on the other hand, are all relatively low in omega-6.

Soybean oil is currently the biggest source of omega-6 fatty acids in the United States because it is really cheap and found in all sorts of processed foods. Because they are cheap, food manufacturers like to also use corn oil, sunflower oil, or safflower oil to make processed food. Baked goods such as cookies and pastries, snack foods like potato chips, ready salad dressings, ready meals, and fast food are almost always made using these oils.

It's also worth noting that very often even many healthy foods can contain vegetable oils. For example, many packaged dried fruits, such as dried cranberries, contain vegetable oils to keep make them shiny and prevent them from sticking. Canned sardines and many granola bars also contain sunflower or other omega-6-rich vegetable oils, so it's crucial to always read the labels.

Nuts and seeds are rich sources of omega-6, but they are whole foods rich in essential minerals such as magnesium, copper, calcium and iron, and have plenty of health benefits. Many grain-based foods also contain significant amounts of omega-6.

ARE THERE OMEGA-6 FATS IN ANIMAL PRODUCTS TOO?

Animal products, too, can contain omega-6 fats. When cows, chickens, or pigs are fed a corn-based diet full of omega-6 fats, these fats enter their meat, eggs, and milk. So when we eat animal fats, their omega-6 to omega-3 ratio reflects what the animals were fed.

Unfortunately, the omega-6 to omega-3 ratios of meat, dairy, and eggs from animals raised on modern feeds are much higher than the ideal 2:1 balance. In contrast, when free-roaming hens feed on insects and green plants, the omega-6 to omega-3 ratio of the eggs they produce is approximately 2:1. Mass-produced commercial eggs can contain as much as twenty times more omega-6 than omega-3.

A study comparing the milks of intensively reared and grass-fed cows in Denmark showed that grass-fed cows produced milk with an omega-6 to omega-3 ratio of 1:1 (having equal amounts of omega-6 and omega-3). By contrast, conventionally grown cows fed a commercial mix of rapeseed, soybean meal, and maize produced milk with an omega-6 to omega-3 ratio of around 5:1.[3]

UNHEALTHY FATS: TRANS FATS

Trans fats rank among the top nutrients on the pro-inflammatory list.

Intake of trans fatty acids, even at low levels (2 percent of total energy intake), is associated with several negative health effects. Increased trans fatty acid intake increases the risk of several chronic diseases, including diabetes, cancer, and stroke.[4]

WHAT ARE TRANS FATS?

Trans fats are produced during the hydrogenation process, when liquid vegetable oils are converted into solid fats by adding hydrogen. The hydrogenated fats become rancid very slowly, and this is the reason why they are widely used by the food industry. They help create products with a much longer shelf life. They also add texture and increase the stability of baked foods, and they save costs for food manufacturers.

Trans, or hydrogenated oils, are most commonly found in margarine, vegetable shortening, packaged snacks, and baked goods (especially premade versions). Trans fats are generally found in cakes, crackers, biscuits, pie crusts, and some cereal bars, so try to keep these snacks to minimum amounts if you cannot avoid them completely. Trans fats are also found in ready-to-use dough and coffee creamers (both dairy and nondairy).

TRANS FATS AND CANCER RISK

The results of the French part of the European Prospective Investigation into Cancer and Nutrition show that high intakes of trans fats are probably one factor contributing to increased risk of invasive breast cancer in women.[5] Other published studies also indicate that a high trans fatty acid intake is associated with increased risk of colorectal and prostate cancers.

Trans fats contribute to systemic inflammation, insulin resistance, and weight gain, all of which are well-known cancer risk factors.

WHAT ABOUT SATURATED FATS?

The facts on saturated fats are a bit different. For many years saturated fats were thought to fuel inflammation and promote cancer. Nowadays this relationship is not so clear.

Recent research shows that a modest proportion of saturated fat in the diet is not harmful, given that the diet is rich in plant foods, olive oil, omega-3 fats, and low-glycemic index carbohydrates (the type of carbohydrates that do not increase blood sugar levels significantly).

One advantage of saturated fats is that they are not oxidized easily when heated. It is for this reason that coconut oil, which is 90 percent saturated, is beginning to be recognized as a good option for cooking oil.[6]

Suggestions:

- Check the labels of the products you buy. Avoid products with hydrogenated or partially hydrogenated oils in their ingredients list.
- Decrease your dependence on packaged foods. Start by eliminating one food group at a time. For example, cook your potatoes from scratch instead of relying on seasoned, boxed versions.
- Try to minimize the intake of ready-made cakes, crackers, biscuits, pie crusts, and some cereal bars.
- Avoid processed and deep-fried foods, as most of them are high in trans fats.

CHAPTER 26

Food Additives Accused of Causing Inflammation

FOOD ADDITIVES ARE SUBSTANCES added to foods to preserve flavor, enhance taste and appearance or prolong shelf-life. With the plethora of processed foods that are being continuously released in the market in recent years, many new additives have been introduced, of both natural and artificial origin. Some of these are controversial with regard to their consequences on health.

CONTROVERSY OVER CARRAGEENAN

One couldn't present the effects of diet on inflammation without reporting on the controversy surrounding carrageenan. Carrageenan is a common food additive that is extracted from red seaweeds. It has no nutritional value and has been used as a thickener and emulsifier for its jelling and stabilizing properties. It is used by the food industry to improve the texture of many common processed foods.

Carrageenan is commonly found in dairy products such as spreadable cheese, flavored milk, sour cream, cottage cheese etc. It is also found in frozen desserts like ice-cream. Carrageenan is often added in non-dairy milks such as almond and soy milk, in coffee creamers and even in nutritional drinks such as some aloe vera juices and supplements. Carrageenan is very commonly used in deli meats and prepackaged foods such as pizzas, dips and even juices.

The FDA insists on the safety of carrageenan despite a number of research studies showing its harmful effects to health. A recent report by the Cornucopia Institute, a corporate and governmental watchdog group, makes a case for banning carrageenan.[1] The report states that experts have known about these adverse effects for decades.

Animal studies have repeatedly shown that food-grade carrageenan causes gastrointestinal inflammation and higher rates of intestinal lesions, ulcerations, and even cancerous tumors.[2]

DEGRADED VERSUS UNDEGRADED CARRAGEENAN

When processed with acid, carrageenan is degraded to a low molecular weight and is called "degraded carrageenan." Degraded carrageenan is such a potent inflammatory agent that it is routinely used by scientists to induce inflammation and other disease in laboratory animals in order to test anti-inflammatory drugs. Degraded carrageenan is not allowed in food.

However, many scientists are concerned that stomach acid can degrade the carrageenan used in foods once it enters the digestive system and expose the intestines to this potent and widely recognized carcinogen.[3] Degraded carrageenan is classified as a "possible human carcinogen" by the International Agency for Research on Cancer.

Carrageenan is used in a very large number of food products. According to Dr. Joanne K. Tobacman, MD, it is easy for the average person to reach doses that are high enough for causing inflammation in the body. Dr. Tobacman, an associate professor of clinical medicine at the University of Illinois College of Medicine, has published over eighteen studies that show that carrageenan is harmful to human health.

Recent studies have found that when laboratory mice were exposed to low concentrations of carrageenan for eighteen days, they developed "profound" glucose intolerance and impaired insulin action, both of which can lead to diabetes.

CARRAGEENAN AND INFLAMMATORY BOWEL DISEASE

Carrageenan has been found to cause colitis in animal models of ulcerative colitis.

According to Dr. Stephen Hanauner, a medical professor and head of gastroenterology and nutrition at the University of Chicago School of Medicine and president of the American College of Gastroenterology since October 2014, "the rising incidence and prevalence of ulcerative colitis across the globe is correlated with the increased consumption of products containing carrageenan".[4]

Many individuals experiencing gastrointestinal symptoms ranging from mild "belly bloat" to irritable bowel syndrome and severe inflammatory bowel disease have noticed that avoiding carrageenan-containing foods leads to significant improvement in their gastrointestinal health. This is why Dr. Stephen Hanauner decided to carry out a controlled clinical trial to investigate the impact of carrageenan on people with inflammatory bowel disease. The results of Dr. Hanauner's study are not out yet, but they are definitely much awaited and will hopefully shed more light on this controversy.

SO WHICH ARE THE FOODS CONTAINING CARRAGEENAN?

Carrageenan can be found in many types of products, including cheese, ice cream, bread, jelly, jam, and most processed meat products such as ham and sliced turkey. It's often used as a stabilizer in beverages whose contents are known to separate, such as chocolate milk and nutritional supplements. It is also used in making almond, soy, and coconut milk. It also may be found in products made with a carrageenan-containing ingredient, such as pies that use condensed milk, although it may not be listed on the product's ingredient list. It doesn't contribute any nutritional value or improve taste, safety, or shelf life.

Surprisingly, carrageenan is also found in products labeled as organic, as the United States Federal organic standards allow nonorganic ingredients to be used for the production of organic products. Carrageenan got approved for use as a nonorganic ingredient in the 1990s.

Suggestions:

- Check the labels of the products you buy and avoid products with carrageenan, especially if you have digestive issues such as abdominal pain, intestinal bloating, spastic colon, irritable bowel syndrome, ulcerative colitis, Crohn's disease or colon cancer.

- Avoid processed and prepackaged food products. Buy whole, natural foods with no additives and foods in their original form (i.e., pure cheese, not processed cheese spreads containing carrageenan).
- Eat meat you can cook rather than processed meat products with carrageenan.

CHAPTER 27

Exposure to Environmental and Dietary Carcinogens

ESTIMATES FROM THE WORLD HEALTH ORGANIZATION and the International Agency for Research on Cancer (IARC) suggest that the fraction of cancers attributable to toxic environmental exposures is between 7 percent and 19 percent.

Official reports, however, such as the United States President's Cancer Panel that was released in 2010, express the fear that the "true burden of environmentally induced cancer has been grossly underestimated".[1] The Panel strongly urged action to reduce people's widespread exposure to carcinogens.

Cancer is caused by changes to certain genes that change the way our cells function. Some of these genetic changes are the result of environmental exposures that damage DNA. These exposures may include substances such as chemicals in tobacco smoke, radiation, and excessive exposure to the ultraviolet rays from the sun. Additionally, our bodies are exposed today to a phenomenal number of environmental toxins ranging from pesticides and herbicides to household chemicals and cleaners, food additives, and perfumes.[2]

The United States permits more than eighty-four thousand chemicals to be used in household products, cosmetics, food, and food packaging, and a majority of these have never been tested for safety. More than ten thousand chemical additives with questionable safety—as most have never been tested in humans—are allowed in food and food packaging alone. Roughly thirteen thousand chemicals are used in cosmetics, of which only 10 percent have been evaluated for safety.[3]

CARCINOGENIC POTENTIAL OF LOW-DOSE EXPOSURES TO CHEMICAL MIXTURES IN THE ENVIRONMENT

A study published in 2015 in the journal *Carcinogenesis* concluded for the first time that even chemicals that are considered to be safe on their own have cumulative effects and act synergistically, resulting in carcinogenic activity. The Halifax Project Task Force that worked on this report involved nearly two hundred scientists from eleven teams of international cancer biologists and toxicologists.[4]

Their analysis found that by acting on various pathways, organs and organ systems, cells, and tissues, the cumulative effects of noncarcinogenic chemicals can act in concert to synergistically produce carcinogenic activity. The amounts of the noncarcinogenic chemicals used in the study are similar to the ones the majority of people are exposed to in today's modern life, and the carcinogenic synergies of these chemicals have been seriously overlooked so far.

The assessment methods used so far have examined the potential risk from single chemicals, so this study opens new roads in assessing the risk from real-life, multiple exposures.

WHAT WE CAN DO

Some cancer-causing exposures are harder to avoid than others, especially if they are in the air we breathe, the water we drink, the food we eat, or the materials we use to do our jobs. Scientists are studying which exposures may cause or contribute to the development of cancer. Understanding which exposures are harmful and are related to cancer and where they are found enables us to avoid or at least reduce them. Unfortunately, it is unrealistic to think you can eliminate all toxins, but you can work to minimize them.

The substances that will be presented in this chapter are among the most likely carcinogens to affect human health. Simply because a substance has been designated as a carcinogen, however, does not mean that it will necessarily cause cancer. Many factors influence whether a person exposed to a carcinogen will develop cancer, including the amount and duration of the exposure and the individual's genetic background.

Suggestions:

- Get a water filter.
- Switch your body care and cleaning products to natural, less harmful alternatives.
- Avoid processed foods. Prepare and cook your food and snacks from fresh, natural ingredients that are free from preservatives, stabilizers, and the like.
- Avoid exposure to plastics and replace plastic containers for food and drinks with glass or stainless steel ones.
- Avoid home fragrances. Replace them with natural essential oils.

AFLATOXINS

Aflatoxins are a family of toxins produced by certain molds such as Aspergillus flavus and Aspergillus parasiticus which grow in soil, decaying vegetation and grains. These molds are often found on agricultural crops such as maize (corn), peanuts, cottonseed, and tree nuts and are abundant in warm and humid regions of the world.

Aflatoxin-producing molds can contaminate crops in the field, at harvest, and during storage, especially following long exposure to high-humidity environment.[5]

HOW ARE WE EXPOSED TO AFLATOXINS?

People can be exposed to aflatoxins by eating contaminated plant products (such as peanuts) or by consuming meat or dairy products from animals that ate contaminated feed. Farmers and other agricultural workers may be exposed by inhaling dust generated during the handling and processing of contaminated crops and feeds.[6]

Aflatoxins are a major health problem mainly in tropical countries, in sub-Saharan countries and south-east Asia such as China.

The most common foods where aflatoxins can be found are peanuts and their products such as peanut butter and corn and its products such as breakfast cereals or pop-corn. Aflatoxins are also found in other nuts and grains including rice, wheat and quinoa, in vegetable oils such as cottonseed oil and soybean oil and in animal products as they enter the food chain via animal feeds.

AFLATOXINS AND LIVER CANCER

Chronic low-level exposure to aflatoxins, particularly aflatoxins B1, is associated with an increased risk of developing impaired immune function and liver cancer.[7]

HOW CAN AFLATOXIN EXPOSURE BE REDUCED?

You can reduce your aflatoxin exposure by discarding nuts that look moldy, discolored, or shriveled. To help minimize risk, governmental authorities in every country such as the U.S. Food and Drug Administration (FDA) test foods that may contain aflatoxins, such as peanuts and peanut butter.

Suggestions:

- Aim for a wide variety of foods in your diet and do not over depend on a few types of foods. Avoid high amounts of corn products and peanuts (including peanut butter).
- Avoid storing your grains and nuts for long periods. Buy them as fresh as you can, and if possible buy local produce to avoid long storage and transfer in conditions where mould might contaminate the products.
- Store your grains, nuts and seeds them in the fridge and do consume them within a couple of months.
- Soaking, sprouting and fermenting grains, beans, legumes, nuts and seeds can reduce mold levels.
- Use detoxifying vegetables and herbs found in chapter 28 regularly, as research has shown they can effectively reduce the carcinogenic effects of aflatoxins.

ARSENIC

Arsenic is one of the world's most toxic elements. It is naturally found in air, water, and soil. It can also be released into the environment by certain agricultural and industrial processes, such as mining and metal smelting. Throughout history, it has been finding its way into our foods. However, this problem is now getting worse as widespread pollution is raising the levels of arsenic in foods, posing a serious health risk.[8]

HOW ARE WE EXPOSED TO ARSENIC?

People may be exposed to arsenic by cigarette smoking, by breathing in other people's smoke (known as secondhand smoke or passive smoking), by drinking contaminated water, or by eating food from plants that were irrigated with contaminated water.

Arsenic comes in two forms, organic and inorganic, with inorganic being more toxic.[9] Inorganic arsenic is naturally present at high levels in the groundwater of certain countries, including the United States.[10] Exposure to arsenic in contaminated drinking water is generally thought to be more harmful to human health than exposure to arsenic in contaminated foods.

Recently, however, studies have detected high levels of arsenic in rice. Rice and rice-based products contain high levels of the inorganic and more toxic form of arsenic. This is a major concern, since rice is a staple food for a large part of the world's population. Also, rice is consumed in large quantities by infants and young children and by people on specific diets, such as gluten- and wheat-free diets.

ARSENIC AND CANCER RISK

The International Agency for Research on Cancer (IARC) has classified arsenic and arsenic compounds as carcinogenic to humans, and has also stated that arsenic in drinking water is carcinogenic to humans.[11]

Prolonged ingestion of arsenic-containing drinking water is associated with an increased risk of bladder cancer. Arsenic exposure is also related to cancers of the skin, lung, digestive tract, liver, kidney, and lymphatic and hematopoietic systems.[12]

Suggestions:

- Avoid cigarette smoke.
- Apply a water filter system to your drinking water.
- Reduce arsenic in your rice by using plenty of water when cooking and by washing the rice in plenty of water before cooking. Research shows that the best way to cook rice for removing most of its stored arsenic is to repeatedly flush it through with fresh hot water.
- Cook your rice as if you were boiling pasta. Ideally increase proportions of water in a ratio of twelve parts water to one part rice. Research has confirmed that arsenic is 'mobile' in liquid water and this method was found to remove up to 57 percent of the grain's arsenic.[13]
- Brown rice contains higher amounts of arsenic than white rice. If you eat large amounts of rice, more than once a day, the white variety may be a better choice.
- Choose aromatic rice, such as basmati or jasmine, as they are lower in arsenic.
- If possible, avoid rice that is grown during the dry season. The use of arsenic-contaminated water is more common during that time.

- Make sure to diversify your diet by eating many different foods. Your diet should never be dominated by one type of food.

BPA

BPA stands for bisphenol A. It is an industrial chemical that has been used to make certain plastics and resins since the 1960s. It is found in polycarbonate plastics and epoxy resins.

Polycarbonate plastics are often used in containers that store food and beverages, such as food containers, water bottles, and baby bottles. Epoxy resins are used to coat the inside of metal products, such as food cans (i.e., soup and tuna cans) and water supply lines.[14] As a component of polycarbonate plastic, over six billion pounds of BPA are produced each year.

BPA, along with other environmental toxins, has been found to mimic estrogens in the human body and to disrupt the normal hormonal functioning of the body (endocrine-disrupting activity).

BPA IN OUR FOOD

Research has shown that BPA can leak into food or beverages from containers that are made with BPA. Detectable amounts can be found in many commercial food products.

We now know that BPA is chronically ingested by humans. Ninety-five percent of adults and children tested in industrialized countries have detectable concentrations of BPA in their urine, which indicates that exposure is both plenty and continuous.[15] BPA has also been measured in the blood of pregnant women, in the blood of embryos, and in amniotic fluid, indicating passage across the placenta.

BPA LINKED TO INCREASED CANCER RISK

In 2012 the U.S. Food and Drug Administration (FDA) said BPA was safe for people of all ages but still banned the use of the chemical in sippy cups, baby bottles, and other containers used by children.

New studies, however, link BPA to numerous conditions, including cancer and obesity.

Research carried out by Kristen Lozada and Ruth Keri at the Case Western Reserve University in Cleveland, Ohio, concluded that exposure to BPA at various time points throughout the life span increases the risk of developing breast cancer in mice.[16] If these mechanisms extend to humans, BPA has the potential to increase susceptibility to breast cancer at low doses if exposure occurs at various important developmental time points. This is strong evidence indicating that fetal exposure to estrogen-mimicking toxins like BPA can causes changes in breast development in childhood that lead to breast cancer manifested during adulthood.

Furthermore, early exposure to BPA increases a person's risk of developing prostate cancer, according to research by Gail Prins, a professor of physiology at the University of Illinois at Chicago. Prins found that BPA's estrogenic effect "reprograms" prostate stem cells, leading to prostate cancer development.[17] The doses of BPA used in her study were similar to those found in previous studies of pregnant American women. "This is the first direct evidence that exposure to BPA during early development, at the levels we see in our day-to-day environment, increases the risk for prostate cancer in human prostate tissue," Prins said in a press release accompanying the research.[18]

Reducing your exposure to BPA is therefore extremely important, especially in women who are planning to become pregnant, are pregnant, or are lactating, and of course in early childhood.

UNEXPECTED SOURCES OF BPA

In 2010 the Environmental Working Group (EWG), an American nonprofit environmental organization that among others specializes in research in the areas of toxic chemicals, conducted tests on major retailers' store receipts and found that 40 percent were coated with BPA.[19] The chemical can rub off on hands or food items. Some may be absorbed through the skin especially of people working as cashiers in these stores.

Suggestions:

- Avoid plastic food and drink containers. Use glass, pyrex, porcelain, ceramic, or stainless steel containers for hot foods and liquids instead.

- Use glass or stainless steel baby bottles.

- Avoid heat for plastic containers. Do not use plastic containers in microwave ovens or in dishwashers, as the plastic may break down over time and allow BPA to leach into foods.

- Avoid completely the use of canned foods, since most cans are lined with BPA-containing resin. Canned food is generally heated to 110 °C (230 °F) during the sterilizing process, resulting in BPA diffusing into the food. Examples are tinned fish, such as tuna and sardines, tinned soups, and tined fruits and vegetables.

- Look for BPA-free products. More and more BPA-free products have come to market. If a product isn't labeled, keep in mind that some, but not all, plastics marked with recycle codes 3 or 7 may be made with BPA.

- According to the United States Environmental Working Group (EWG), you can reduce exposure to BPA by saying no to receipts when possible and by washing your hands before preparing and eating food after handling receipts. This might be especially useful when eating out, when eating a snack you just bought and so on.

- The EWG also advices to never give children a receipt to hold or play with and not to recycle receipts and other thermal paper, as BPA residues will contaminate recycled paper.

PHTHALATES

Phthalates are another group of chemicals that are known hormone disruptors. They are commonly used to make plastics soft and flexible. They are found in a wide variety of common products, including plastics, cosmetics such as nail polishes and perfumes, pharmaceuticals, and baby care products. They are also found in building materials, modeling clay, automobiles, cleaning materials, and insecticides.

Phthalates from cosmetics are easily absorbed through the skin and can also enter the body through inhalation and through food. Food packaging is one of the major sources of some phthalates, as phthalates in plastic packaging leach into the food inside.

THE HEALTH RISKS OF PHTHALATES

Research on phthalates and cancer in humans is very limited, but there is a probable link. There have been small studies linking phthalates to premenopausal breast cancer risk but more research needs to be done to clarify the phthalate to cancer risk.[20] The International Agency for Research on Cancer (IARC) classifies diethylhexyl phthalate (DEHP), a type of phthalate, as a possible cause of cancer.[21]

Other studies have linked phthalates to hormone changes, lower sperm count, less mobile sperm, birth defects in the male reproductive system, obesity, diabetes, and thyroid irregularities.

Suggestions:

- Minimize fatty foods exposed to flexible plastics such as cheese, butter, and pies.

- Look for plastic products marked "phthalate-free" or "PVC-free" and avoid plastics with recycling code no. 3.

- Avoid household cleaners and cosmetics with "fragrance" on the label.

- Avoid plastic food containers and plastic wrap (especially those labeled no. 3). Replace with glass or stainless steel ones.

- Never heat your food in plastic.

- Avoid children's plastic toys as much as possible (some phthalates are already banned in kids' products).

- Look for fragrance-free products. One artificial fragrance can contain hundreds of potentially toxic chemicals.

- Switch over to organic natural toiletries, including shampoo, toothpaste, antiperspirants, and cosmetics.

- The Environmental Working Group's Skin Deep database can help you find personal care products that are free of phthalates and other potentially dangerous chemicals. You can access it here : http://www.ewg.org/skindeep/

NONSTICK COOKWARE

Nonstick cookware has received a lot of bad publicity over its potential health risks. Nonstick cookware refers to cookware that has a chemical coating so that food doesn't stick.[22]

There is a big variety of nonstick pans, pots and casseroles in the market. The chemical used for the production of nonstick cookware is also found in stain-resistant carpets, and even in the lining of microwave popcorn bags.

The potentially harmful ingredient in nonstick cookware is PFOA (perfluorooctanoic acid). PFOA is so widespread and so extraordinarily persistent that it is found in the blood of 99 percent of Americans.

PFOA IN NONSTICK COOKWARE AND CANCER RISK

Data from animal studies show that PFOA can cause several types of cancer and may have toxic effects on the immune, liver, and endocrine systems.[23] However, human studies on PFOA are very limited.

The US Environmental Protection Agency's (EPA's) Scientific Advisory Board released a draft report in 2006 on PFOA. It stated that there is "suggestive evidence of carcinogenicity, but not sufficient to assess human carcinogenic potential." The board agreed that new evidence would be considered as it becomes available.[24]

However, new data have become available since then, the most important being the report of a panel of three epidemiologists known as C8. This expert panel was appointed by the Circuit Court of Wood County following a lawsuit against a company for contaminating groundwater with PFOA over several decades.[25]

The official report of the panel that was released in April 2012 titled "Probable link evaluation of cancer", stated that, "on the basis of epidemiologic and other data available to the C8 Science Panel, we conclude that there is a probable link between exposure to PFOA and testicular and kidney cancer." The C8 Science Panel also concluded that PFOA was also probably linked to ulcerative colitis, thyroid disease, hypercholesterolemia, and pregnancy-induced hypertension.[26]

Suggestions:

- Avoid nonstick cookware.
- Avoid stain- and water-resistant coatings on clothing, furniture, and carpets.

DIOXINS

Dioxins are a group of highly toxic chemicals. They are not created intentionally, but are produced as a result of human activities like the burning of trash and the burning of products containing PVC, PCBs, and other chlorinated compounds. Dioxins are also formed during the production of certain herbicides and by certain industrial processes that use chlorine, such as the bleaching of pulp paper with free chlorine, and the combustion of diesel and gasoline. Dioxins might also be released in the environment as a result of natural processes like forest fires.[27, 28, 29]

Dioxins are very persistent pollutants. They take a very long time to break down once they are released in the environment.

DIOXINS IN THE ENVIRONMENT, IN OUR FOOD AND IN OUR BODIES

Dioxins are found throughout the world in the environment. They enter the food chain as they fall on field crops through the air, then they get eaten by farm animals through their feed or enter waters from which seafood is caught.

They accumulate in the fat of animals and bioaccumulate up the food chain. More than 90 percent of human exposure is through fatty food of animal origin, mainly meat and dairy products, fish, and shellfish, and through breast milk.

There is much variation between different countries as to the most important foods contributing to dioxin intake. In the United States and Central Europe, milk, dairy products, and meat have been by far the most important sources. In some countries, notably in the Scandinavian region, fish is the most important source. In most countries, a significant decrease in dioxin intake has occurred due to stricter controls on dioxin release by industry set during the last twenty years.[30]

In humans, dioxins leave the body at a very slow pace. It has been estimated that it takes seven to eleven years for dioxin levels to drop by half.

In 2001, a United Nations environmental treaty was signed by the European Union and 178 other UN member states. The so-called Stockholm Convention on Persistent Organic Pollutants banned the production of a number of intentionally produced pollutants such as dioxins.[31] Dioxins are also no longer produced in the United States.

Research published in 2010 by the Environmental Protection Agency in the United States has shown that as a result of numerous regulatory actions taken by governments throughout the world, dioxin levels in the food supply and in the environment have been declining over the past three decades.[32] Yet, because the chemicals are persistent and bioaccumulate, most people in the developed countries still have substantial levels of dioxins in their bodies. The most recent data in studies of Americans indicate that over 95 percent have measurable levels of dioxins in their bodies.

THE TOXIC EFFECTS OF DIOXINS ON HUMAN HEALTH

Dioxins are highly toxic and are powerful human carcinogens. In 1997 the International Agency for Research on Cancer classified the most potent dioxin (TCDD) as a known human carcinogen. Three years later, in 2000, the U.S. Environmental Protection Agency also officially declared TCDD to be a known carcinogen.[33]

Dioxins are also endocrine disruptors. They disrupt the delicate ways that both male and female sex hormone signaling occurs in the body. Recent research has shown that exposure to low levels of dioxins in utero and early in life can permanently affect sperm quality and lower the sperm count in men during their prime reproductive years.

Dioxins also damage the immune system and lead to developmental problems.

HIGH AMOUNTS OF DIOXINS IN FARMED VERSUS WILD SALMON

As a result of environmental pollution, dioxins, PCBs, and other pollutants have been poured into the oceans and eventually bioaccumulate in fish.

In early 2000, a number of studies found that concentrations of dioxins, PCBs, and pesticides were significantly higher in farm-raised salmon than in wild Pacific salmon. Also, salmon raised in European farms were found to have significantly higher contaminant concentrations than salmon raised on North and South American farms.[34]

The same studies also suggested that cancer risk to humans was higher with even low levels of consumption of farmed salmon as compared to similar quantities of wild salmon. The US Environmental Protection Agency (EPA) recommends that consumption of farmed salmon be restricted to approximately once per month.

The semi-enclosed Baltic Sea, surrounded by highly industrialized countries, is considered to be one of the most contaminated environments in the world. Since 2002, Swedish authorities have been required by law to inform consumers about dangerous dioxins found in Swedish salmon. Exporting Baltic Sea salmon to other European Union member states was also banned at the time.[35]

The 2002 laws came about after the EU introduced rules on how much dioxin is permissible in different foods. The EU, however, issued an exemption for sales in Sweden, as long as its authorities made an effort to inform the public about potential health risks.

One such guideline was to warn pregnant women and children not to eat Baltic Sea salmon more than two or three times a year. Yet while restrictions are in place, fishermen have continued to pull up large numbers of salmon from the Baltic Sea. In 2012, an estimated 250 tons of salmon were fished in Sweden alone. Recent news reports from the BBC News and other news agencies suggest that Swedish salmon sales 'breached EU ban" over dioxins and exported illegally large volumes of salmon to neighboring EU countries like France, Denmark and the Netherlands. This resulted in Swedish salmon ending up in supermarket aisles and on restaurant plates in Europe without the dioxin warning.[36, 37]

More recent studies, such as one by Ole Jakob Nostbakken and his team published in 2015 in the journal *Environment International*, have found that levels of contaminants in Norwegian farmed salmon have decreased from 1999 to 2011.[38] Even with these reported reductions in dioxin levels in Norwegian salmon, however, there are reports that question the safety of dioxin levels of farmed salmon. Some consumer groups even claim that dioxin levels are still seven times higher than the WHO safe limits for toxin exposure.[39]

Suggestions:

- Dioxins are stored in the fat of animals, so limit your consumption of protein sources that are high in animal fat, such as meats and high-fat dairy products such as milk, eggs, cheese, and butter.
- Eat fewer animal products.
- Instead of eating farm-raised fish, which are often heavily contaminated with PCBs and dioxins, eat fish that is wild-caught and lab tested for purity, such as wild-caught Alaskan salmon. Alternatively, you can supplement with a high-quality krill oil or omega-3 supplement that has been distilled to remove environmental toxins.

PESTICIDES

Pesticides are a group of many different toxic chemicals. They are toxic in nature, as they are released intentionally into the environment to kill living organisms such as insects (insecticides), plants (herbicides), and fungi (fungicides) that are considered as "pests".

PESTICIDES AND HEALTH RISKS

Many pesticides pose health dangers to people. As acknowledged by U.S. and international government agencies, different pesticides have been linked to a variety of health problems, including brain and nervous system toxicity, cancer, hormone disruption, attention deficit hyperactivity disorder (ADHD), and skin, eye and lung irritation.[40]

Studies show that there may be a connection between pesticide exposure and cancer in adults and children. According to the Canadian Cancer Society, research does not show a definite link between most of the pesticides studied and human cancer. It does, however, suggest a possible connection with cancers such as non-Hodgkin lymphoma, multiple myeloma, chronic lymphocytic leukemia, and prostate, testicular, pancreatic, lung, and non-melanoma skin cancers. Studies of pesticides and childhood cancer show a possible connection with leukemia and non-Hodgkin lymphoma.[41]

Until more clear knowledge is available on how pesticides affect our health and possible cancer risk, it would be wise to take a few steps to minimize one's exposure to pesticide residues on our food.

WHICH FOODS ARE THE WORST FOR PESTICIDE RESIDUES

The Environmental Working Group (EWG), a nonprofit United States organization dedicated to protecting human health and the environment, releases a yearly list of the most pesticide-loaded fruits and vegetables, known as the Dirty Dozen list.[42] The EWG shopper's guide as it is called is based on laboratory tests done on thousands of fruits and vegetables as they are typically eaten. This means that they are washed and, when applicable, peeled before they are tested.

For years non-organic apples topped the list but in 2016 strawberries appeared to have the highest pesticide load. One of the key findings of the Dirty Dozen list for 2016 is that single samples of strawberries showed seventeen different pesticides. Strawberries are followed by apples, nectarines, peaches, celery, grapes, cherries, spinach, tomatoes, sweet bell peppers, cherry tomatoes, and cucumbers.

The EWG also releases the Clean Fifteen list, a yearly list that contains produce with the least types on pesticides and with low total concentrations of pesticides. The list for 2016 consisted of avocados, sweet corn, pineapples, cabbage, frozen sweet peas, onions, asparagus, mangoes, papayas, kiwis, eggplant, honeydew melon, grapefruit, cantaloupe, and cauliflower. Avocados were the cleanest in the list, as only 1 percent of avocado samples showed any detectable pesticides.

Multiple pesticide residues are extremely rare on Clean Fifteen vegetables. Only 5 percent of Clean Fifteen samples had two or more pesticides and no single fruit sample from the Clean Fifteen list tested positive for more than four types of pesticides. On the contrary, some fruits and vegetables in the Dirty Dozen list tested positive for fifteen and more types of pesticides.

Suggestions:

- Wash all fresh vegetables and fruit thoroughly with lots of running water.
- Wash your fruit and vegetables in a bowl of water with two to three tablespoons of vinegar. Let them soak in it for about ten minutes.

- Use a small scrub brush to clean the skin of vegetables and fruit if the skin will be eaten, for example, apples, potatoes, and cucumbers.
- Peel off the outer skin of vegetables and fruit. Trim the outer leaves of leafy vegetables, and then wash thoroughly.
- If possible, choose organically grown fruits and vegetables.
- Consider buying the fruits and vegetables found in the yearly Dirty Dozen list from organic producers. If this is not possible or is very costly for your family, replace them with fruits and vegetables from the Clean Fifteen list.

CHLORINATED WATER

Chlorinated water is water with chlorine added to it. Chlorine is added to disinfect the water and make it suitable for drinking by killing bacteria and other microbes in untreated water. When chlorine interacts with organic matter (such as dead leaves and soil) in untreated water, it forms new chemicals that remain in the water. These are called chlorination by-products, which are believed to increase cancer risk.

The International Agency for Research on Cancer (IARC) classifies some chlorination by-products as possible causes of cancer. For decades, researchers have studied the long-term effects of using chlorinated tap water. Most studies have shown that when people are exposed to chlorinated water over long periods of time, it slightly increases the risk of bladder cancer. Some studies have also found links to colorectal cancer, but we need more research to be sure of this link.[43] Animal studies have also shown that two of the most common chlorination by-products can cause cancer in laboratory animals.

Suggestions:

- Use devices that filter your home's drinking water and if possible all the water in your house. Make sure your filters are certified with international foundations' standards and change the filters according to the manufacturer's instructions.

ALCOHOL

Alcoholic beverages have been produced and consumed by humans since pre-historic times. Alcohol is used at social events and occasions as a symbol of celebration, friendship and having a good time. Most people drink alcohol for socializing. Others drink alcohol to feel more relaxed and at ease, while a minority of people often drink alcohol in order to get drunk and lose their inhibitions.

Alcohol intake can lead to dependence and long term alcohol overuse can lead to serious health effects such as depression, anxiety, mood swings, high blood pressure, liver disease and high blood lipids.

Excessive alcohol intake has been found in scientific studies to increase cancer risk.[44] According to Cancer Research UK and the American Cancer Society, alcohol can increase the risk of a number of cancers, such as mouth, liver, breast, bowel, and throat cancer.[45, 46]

DIET QUALITY INFLUENCES THE EFFECT OF ALCOHOL ON CANCER RISK

According to Dr. David Servan-Schreiber in his bestselling book *Anticancer—A New Way of Life*, the dietary context in which alcohol is consumed can considerably modify the body's response to alcohol.[47] For example, when the intake of omega-6 to omega-3 fatty acids is unbalanced with an excess of omega-6 in the diet, the carcinogenic free radicals produced with the consumption of alcohol increase by a factor of five to ten.

Also, studies have shown that breast cancer risk in women was increased by alcohol only in those women who had a low intake of green vegetables, resulting in a low folate intake. In relation to breast cancer, studies have found that alcohol increases the level of estrogen in the body. High levels of estrogen are known to encourage the development of breast cancer. It has been found that when drinking alcohol on a daily basis, each unit of alcohol increases the risk of breast cancer by 7 percent to 11 percent.

WHAT ABOUT THE PROTECTIVE EFFECT OF RESVERATROL IN RED WINE?

As analyzed earlier in the book, resveratrol, one of the substances in red wine, has been extensively studied for its anticancer properties. The reported protective effect of red wine is significantly enhanced when it is consumed in the context of a healthy and balanced diet, especially as part of the Mediterranean diet. The main characteristics of this diet are the plentiful colored vegetables rich in polyphenols, flavonoids, beta-carotenes, and folates and the high fish intake, leading to a better balance of omega-3 to omega-6 fatty acids.

Suggestions:

- The more you cut down alcohol, the more you cut your cancer risk.
- If you drink alcohol, limit your intake to no more than one to two drinks per day for men and one drink a day for women.

Toxin Removal and Physical Activity

CHAPTER 28

Enhance Your Ability to Remove Toxins

TOXINS SLOWLY DAMAGE OUR HEALTH

The world around us is not as clean and pure as it once was. Toxic metals are present in the environment at levels which are much higher than ever before. Toxic chemicals, heavy metals, and toxins from cigarette smoking, excessive alcohol consumption, and indoor and outdoor pollution enter the body constantly. They might enter through the air we breathe, the water we drink, the food we eat, or the personal care products we choose.

Chemicals such as pesticides, chlorine, dioxins, PCBs, and acrylamide build up over time, gradually leading to a number of diseases and notably increasing cancer risk.

Various heavy metals are commonly ingested through the food that we eat, even though the Environmental Protection Agency warns that there is no safe level for any heavy metal in the body. Toxic metals commonly stored in the body at high concentrations are arsenic, cadmium, lead and mercury.

Toxins can slowly damage cells, tissues, organs and systems in the body. They interfere with normal hormonal function, increase free radical damage, and lead to chronic health problems. When the body is exposed to high levels of toxins, the immune system becomes weakened and consequently fails to protect the body. Heavy metal toxicity has serious health effects, ranging from brain fog and depression to heart disease, Alzheimer's and even cancer.

THE NEED FOR DETOXIFYING THE BODY

Various organs in the body are naturally designed to eliminate toxins. These are the lymphatic system, the large intestine, the kidneys, the skin, and the lungs.

Very often some of the toxin removal canals become blocked, as in the case of constipation. Constipation is often related to the leaky gut syndrome. In leaky gut syndrome, the thin lining of the intestinal wall becomes permeable and allows toxins that should have been excreted from the gut to enter the blood. This eventually results in toxins and undigested molecules to enter the bloodstream and harm the body in various ways.

In the modern world in which most of us live today, the exposure to man-made toxic chemicals is higher than even before. When the toxins entering the body exceed its natural detoxification capacity, the liver's detoxification system is overloaded. The continuous cleaning process can exhaust organs such as the liver and result in impaired toxin removal and in high levels of toxins accumulating in the body.

This is the reason why, over a period of time, the body's detox organs need to be detoxified. Detoxing and cleansing your body of toxins periodically can help counteract some of the damage caused by the various toxins mentioned above.

People living stressful and hectic lifestyles, people who often feel tired and over worked, and those having various hormonal issues would greatly benefit from a cleanse or detoxification program. Regular intake of ready meals and packaged foods, common food cravings and overindulge in food and drink, are also indications that one would greatly benefit from such programs.

A cleanse or detoxification program is designed to optimize the elimination of toxins from the body and cleanse the digestive system. It can re-boot and rebalance your body and ensure optimal functioning of each organ. It can increase your vitality, promote good health, support a healthy immune system and protect the body from premature ageing.

ENHANCE YOUR ABILITY TO REMOVE TOXINS

The Detoxification Process

In the past the idea of detoxing was restricted to fasting and to keeping nutritional intake to a minimum. Yet now we know better. Even though the body has the ability to neutralize and excrete dangerous toxins, we can aid the difficult tasks of detoxification by taking some extra measures and by adding specific foods and nutrients to our diet.

In order to enhance the body's ability to remove toxins, one has to build a good functioning gut, optimize liver function and follow some basic detoxing strategies. These strategies involve following a supervised detox or cleanse diet once or twice a year and adding foods and herbs with detoxing powers in our daily routine.

A. Build a Good-Functioning Gut

Even if the liver is working at its best and keeps on throwing neutralized toxins to the intestines, if the large intestine is not working properly, then the toxins will build up locally and cause harm. So before you consider steps to support your liver, the first step for ensuring proper toxin removal from the body is to have a good-functioning gut. When this is achieved, then you can move on and repair the filters of your system, which are the liver, the lymphatic system, and the kidneys.

Step 1: Change Your Diet

Start with a change in your diet. Most people's diets today are low in fruits and vegetables, fiber, and water. This leads to constipation. Improving the diet can solve the problem for most people.

Add Fiber

At your two main meals aim to fill at least half of your plate with salads and cooked and raw vegetables. Concentrate on eating more fiber by eating the skin of the fruits, eating the skin of the potatoes, and choosing whole-grain rice. However, if your fresh produce is not organic, it is better to take the skin off.

Rehydrate

One of the main reasons why so many people today are constipated is dehydration. Change your daily routine and try to have water always available to you. Drinking more water will stimulate the natural peristaltic movement of the colon, leading it to function normally. It will flush out the harmful toxins and keep the body hydrated.

Don't count on your thirst to guide your water intake, rather make a good hydration plan and stick to it. Build your intake gradually and aim to reach eight to ten glasses of water per day. Fresh fruit, vegetable juices, herbal teas, and liquid foods also hydrate you.

Add Seeds

Unprocessed foods such as fresh fruits and vegetables, and in particular the seeds they contain, have a very high toxin-capturing capacity. Strawberries, which are full of small seeds in their outer part, have the capacity to bind 90 percent of dietary mercury. Also, fruit seeds in general were found to be very effective in binding and removing arsenic and carrying it out of the body. Seeds like chia seeds and flaxseeds work miracles in establishing a regular bowel opening and cleaning the gut.

Step 2: Establish a Good Exercise Routine

The bowel is a muscle tube, and like all the muscles in our body, it works better when we exercise. Walking thirty minutes a day or doing other activities can help in establishing a regular bowel movement.

Step 3: Build a Healthy Bacterial Balance

Our intestines are the home for billions of bacteria. Beneficial bacteria play a key role in the immune system and in regulating the detoxification of the intestines. Probiotics are foods or supplements that replenish the good bacteria in the gut. One can get probiotics from everyday foods, like authentic yogurt, kefir, and fermented foods like miso, sauerkraut, and fermented vegetables. Very often it is beneficial to take a supplement of beneficial bacteria to restore gut balance more quickly.

Certain strains of probiotic bacteria can minimize toxin exposure by trapping and metabolizing toxic chemicals or heavy metals.[1] Additionally, the production of the short-chain fatty acid butyrate by lactic acid bacteria (from the fermentation of dietary fiber) has been shown to stimulate the production of some of the main detoxifying enzymes in the intestines. This may also contribute to some of the anticarcinogenic properties of dietary fiber.

Step 4: Consider Herbal Detoxification Products

Those who follow Steps 1, 2, and 3 and still don't have regular bowel movements should consider using some herbal remedies. Aloe, cascara sagrada, senna, and slippery elm are among the most common herbs used for treating constipation.

B. Optimize Liver Function

The liver is the second-largest organ in the body. Apart from playing a central role in metabolism, its other main function is detoxification. The liver does the extraordinary job of protecting us from the damaging effects of the numerous toxic compounds to which we are exposed daily.

The liver has a key role in the detoxifying processes of the body. Toxic chemicals constantly challenge the liver as the blood passes through to be filtered. In the liver these toxins become neutralized and are converted to compounds that can then be flushed out in the urine or feces.

There are three main detoxification steps or pathways in the liver. The first involves filtering the blood to remove large toxins, and the second involves a two-step enzymatic process for breaking down and neutralizing toxins. The last step involves the actual excretion of the toxins from the body through the synthesis and secretion of bile.

As the liver breaks down and neutralizes toxins, free radicals are formed.[2] Excessive production of free radicals is one of the most common causes of liver damage. An adequate supply of antioxidants is essential in any program designed to protect and detox the liver.

Step 1: Ensure Optimal Glutathione Levels

The most important antioxidant for neutralizing the free radicals that are formed within the liver is glutathione peroxidase. This strong antioxidant molecule is naturally produced in the liver. Exposure to high levels of toxins and heavy metals can deplete it faster than it can be replenished.

Glutathione is often given as an injection to patients receiving chemotherapy to prevent some of its toxic side effects. Glutathione supplementation can enhance the liver's natural antioxidant capacity and enhance its ability to detoxify safely. Glutathione supplementation however needs to be done under the supervision of a trained health care professional. If taken orally it gets digested and inactivated, so your health care provider can assist in identifying the most appropriate method of administration for your case.

Glutathione activity greatly depends on the trace element selenium. Selenium deficiency has been linked to low glutathione levels. Research has shown that boosting selenium intake improves the antioxidant activity within the liver.

Selenium is known to detoxify liver enzymes, to act as an anti-inflammatory factor within the body, and to amplify the body's antioxidant defense. Scientific evidence has proven that adequate selenium levels can cut cancer risk and even help in slowing down existing cancer's progression and tumor growth.[3]

Just one or two Brazil nuts a day can give you all the selenium you need for your day, which is 200 µg. Studies have shown that 200 µg of selenium can be effective in protecting the DNA, reducing the risk for cell mutation and cancer development.

Step 2: Use Milk Thistle

Milk Thistle is a plant used by herbalists for many centuries to treat various liver disorders, as it stimulates the growth and regeneration of injured liver cells. This first-class herb protects the liver against chemical toxicity. It stimulates phase I and phase II detoxification pathways and can be particularly effective both for cancer prevention and for helping while undergoing chemotherapy or taking other toxic medication.

Silymarin, the active component of milk thistle, has proven to be one of the most potent liver-protecting substances. Milk thistle is approved for use in liver damage, as it has been found to stimulate the synthesis of new liver cells to replace the older, damaged ones.[4]

Using milk thistle for a few weeks, a few times per year can be particularly beneficial for people who drink alcohol regularly, who often indulge in high fat meals, who have high blood lipid levels, and who take medications regularly.

A number of studies have established a protective role of milk thistle in cancer. Silymarin has been found to regulate the imbalance between cell survival and cell death (apoptosis). In addition, it has been shown to have anti-inflammatory as well as anti-metastatic activity.

Cancer patients can combine their therapies with milk thistle to prevent or reduce chemotherapy- and radiotherapy-induced toxicity.[5]

C. Help your Body Eliminate Toxins by Following a Detox Program

Detoxification or "cleaning" diets are short-term interventions designed to eliminate toxins from the body and promote health. Generally, a detoxification or "detox" diet aims to minimize the amount of chemicals and stressors entering the body and to stimulate the body's detoxification processes. Cleanse or detox diets also contain foods or herbal supplements that help in the elimination of toxins from the body.[6]

Detox diets are often laughed at by the medical community. The truth is that they have not been studied in depth by well-controlled and large enough studies. People who follow various detox plans often report improved energy, clearer skin, improvements in bowel movements, improved digestion, and increased concentration after a detox diet.

Detox diets range from total starvation, water-only fasts, to juice fasts and food modification approaches that often involve the use of specific nutrient supplements, herbs, or super foods.

The type of detox plan that best suits your needs depends on your personal health circumstances and goals. If a person has been through chemotherapy, for example, an intense period of detoxification through water fasting could cause damage to the kidneys. Also, people who are ill should be very careful about doing any kind of detox, as this might deteriorate their health even further, making them more sick.

In such cases, a mild approach to detox would be more appropriate, and the guidance of a trained health care provider is necessary. Very often people experience side effects from detoxing, such as headaches, uncomfortable bowel movements, flatulence, fatigue, and lethargy.

Experts in the field advise that people should use caution and evaluate their current state of health before beginning any kind of detoxification program.

A detox needs to be started gradually. There are some priorities that have to be taken into account before starting a detox. First, one has to improve one's diet and lifestyle, have access to clean, filtered water, ensure optimum organ support, and perhaps use specific organ-stimulating supplements. For example, one cannot start a liver detox if one has chronic constipation. Constipation has to be addressed first before considering proceeding to a detox.

BASIC DETOX NUTRITIONAL TOOLS

A number of nutritional strategies, foods, herbs, and super foods can be used for aiding the detoxification of the body.

Fruits and Vegetables are Key Components of Detox Plans

There is evidence that many components of common fruits and vegetables are useful in eliminating toxic metals from the body. For example, coriander, malic acid (found in grapes), citric acid (found in citrus fruits), succinic acid (found in apples and blueberries), pectins (found in apples and in the peel and pulp of citrus fruits), and chlorella (a type of green algae) have natural chelating properties, suggesting that they are useful for the elimination of toxic metals.[7] Fruits and vegetables also help by making the body more alkaline, helping the body maintain its optimal acid/alkaline balance.

Artichoke

This edible flower is rich in liver protective ingredients, including cynarin, a compound that stimulates liver and gallbladder function. Artichokes can protect and regenerate the liver and protect the body against many detrimental toxins. They also support kidney function. Artichokes protect livers' glutathione levels from destruction from various oxidative agents.

Beetroot

Fresh beetroot is your liver's best friend. It's vibrant, purple-red color, is due to betalains, phytonutrients that have anti-inflammatory properties. Beetroots are among the richest sources of betaine, an amino acid that is associated with liver detoxification. Betaine helps the liver break down fats which are then thrown into the small intestine in the form of bile. It has been particularly studied for its ability to prevent and reverse liver damage caused by excessive alcohol intake. Beetroots have also been found to protect the liver from various toxic substances such as some prescription medications and pesticides.

Broccoli

Broccoli improves the phase 2 detoxification pathway on the liver by increasing Glutathione-S-Transferase.

Artichoke

This edible flower is rich in liver protective ingredients, including cynarin, a compound that stimulates liver and gallbladder. Artichokes can protect and regenerate the liver and protect the body against many detrimental toxins. They also support kidney function. Artichokes protect the livers' glutathione levels from destruction from various oxidative agents.

Coriander Leaf

Traditionally coriander has been known for its ability to stimulate digestion as well as calm the intestinal tract and strengthen the stomach and its secretions. Studies have shown that coriander leaves may assist in the removal of the heavy metals aluminium, lead, and mercury from the body.[8,9]

Garlic

Garlic is an excellent detoxification aid. It encourages production of the potent detoxifying antioxidant glutathione.

Lemon

Squeezing a lemon in water every day is a very common thing to do among people who want a gentle daily detox aid. Lemons are known to excrete toxins away from the liver. D-limonene from citrus oil has been shown to increase the activity of phase I and II detoxifying enzymes.[10] These enzymes act in either the intestines or liver by metabolizing clinical drugs and several environmental toxins into water-soluble substances that can be excreted from the body.

A study of Korean overweight women showed that those participants who followed a lemon detox program had a significant body fat reduction accompanied by some detoxic effects related to decreased levels of serum CRP (an indicator of inflammation).[11]

Chlorella and Spirulina

Spirulina and chlorella are well-known detoxifying agents. They are able to bind and remove heavy metals such as aluminum, mercury, cadmium, and arsenic from the body. From animal studies we know that chlorella can also to help with the elimination of some pesticides, PCBs, and dioxins.[12]

Chlorella is a single-cell green algae that contains the green photosynthetic pigment chlorophyll. The unique chemical structure of chlorophyll enables it to bind and "trap" toxins in the gut, preventing their absorption. In animal models chlorophyll and its derivative chlorophyllin lower the bioavailability and accelerate the excretion of several environmental carcinogens.

In a human study, DNA damage was reduced by 55 percent in the people taking chlorophyllin three times a day as compared to controls. This was a very significant result, as the study was done in Qidong, an area in China with a high incidence of liver cancer due to exposure to aflatoxin (a toxin produced by a species of the fungus Aspergillus).[13]

Wheat Leaf Powder, Barley Leaf Powder, Spinach Leaf, and Alfalfa Herb Powder

All these green leaf powders are rich super antioxidant foods. All of them are rich in natural vitamin C and B group vitamins, beta-carotene, potassium, calcium, and magnesium. Like chlorella, they also contain large amounts of chlorophyll, which acts as a very powerful antioxidant. These powders are high in essential nutrients and play a unique role in boosting your health and vitality.

Suggestions:

- Make sure you maintain a healthy digestive system by having a high fiber diet with a lot of fruit and vegetables, exercising regularly and drinking a lot of clean water.

- If you have constipation take the steps outlined in this chapter to overcome it.

- Add probiotic foods in your diet such as kefir, authentic yogurt, miso, sauerkraut and fermented vegetables.

- Eat a couple of Brazil nuts a day for maintaining a regular intake of selenium, a mineral that stimulates glutathione, the most potent liver antioxidant that neutralizes free radicals and dangerous toxins.

- Consider supplementing with milk thistle for a few weeks, a few times per year, to enable the best functioning of your liver.

- Eat frequently foods and herbs that have detoxing powers, such as broccoli, beetroots, artichokes, garlic, lemon and coriander.

- Follow a supervised detox or cleansing program once or twice per year to ensure optimal elimination of toxins and for giving a helping hand to your toxin elimination organs.

CHAPTER 29

Physical Activity: A Powerful Weapon against Cancer

THE LINK BETWEEN EXERCISE AND CANCER has been the subject of numerous studies. All studies have shown consistent evidence that moderate to vigorous physical activity can lower cancer risk. The results have been stronger for cancers of the breast, colon, endometrium, and prostate.[1,2,3]

Not only is exercise able to prevent cancer but today many oncologists encourage their patients to start or continue exercising while doing their cancer treatments. Physical activity is advised for cancer patients, as a growing body of evidence suggests that exercise after a cancer diagnosis can significantly decrease the risk of cancer progression, prevent cancer recurrence, and increase survival. Numerous research studies have also shown that being active can reduce treatment-related side effects and improve cancer patients' quality of life.[4,5]

EXERCISE SUPPORTS THE LYMPHATIC SYSTEM

Exercise is among the best techniques for detoxing the body, as it ensures that the lymphatic system flows properly. The lymphatic system is the body's metabolic waste disposal system as it clears away toxins from the cells. It consists of ducts and channels which flow all over your body. Waste products of the metabolism of each cell and unwanted toxics travel through the lymph, from tiny lymphatic tubules into larger lymphatic vessels, eventually reaching the lymph ducts. There, they get filtered, and the toxins are sent to the liver and kidneys for excretion.

Unlike vessels of the circulatory system, the lymph vessels are not equipped with surrounding muscles, nor are they powered by the action of the heart muscles. Instead, the lymphatic system depends entirely upon gravity, and on the action of the muscles of the body in order to flow properly. By simply walking you are actually enabling lymphatic fluid to flow through the body. One of the best exercises for helping lymphatic flow is hopping on a trampoline.

EXERCISE IMPROVES OVERALL HEALTH STATUS

Physical activity acts in a variety of ways to reduce cancer risk. It helps maintain a healthy body weight by balancing caloric intake with energy expenditure, and may help to prevent certain cancers both directly and indirectly. A physically active lifestyle also protects from other chronic diseases, such as heart disease, diabetes, and osteoporosis.[6]

Exercise improves the physical fitness of the body, which means a better aerobic capacity, increased strength, and improved flexibility. As reported in the US Physical Activity Guidelines, exercise also enhances brain function and improves the body's response to the stresses of disease and aging.[7]

Exercising also reduces the amount of fat stored in the body. As in animals and fish, our body fat is the main storage site for potentially carcinogenic environmental toxins. So when we enhance the body's capacity to burn fat by exercising, at the same time, we enable it to remove stored toxins. Of course, for this to happen efficiently, we need to first ensure that our detox channels are open by having regular bowel activity, eating a high-fiber diet, and drinking a lot of clean water.

Exercise also improves the body's hormonal balance. It reduces the excess estrogens and testosterone that are related to cancers of the breast, ovary, uterus, prostate, and testicles.

Furthermore, exercise improves blood sugar control and as a result insulin and insulin growth factor are reduced.[8] As discussed in the first chapters of the book, high blood sugar, high insulin levels, and IGF are related to inflammation and increased cancer risk, so exercise protects the body indirectly by improving sugar metabolism.[9]

Exercise has a direct, positive effect on the immune system. A review of twenty-one studies on the effects of exercise on immune function in patients with cancer found strong evidence to suggest that the natural killer cells (NK) increase and become more efficient after exercising. Natural killer cells are part of our first line of defense against cancer. They are lymphocytes able to bind and kill certain cancer cells.[10]

Last but not least, we have to acknowledge the effect of exercise on improving our psychological balance. Exercise enhances mood and creates a feeling of being positive, creative, and energetic. It creates a feeling that we are connected with our bodies and it boosts determination to proceed with positive changes in life. Exercise has also been shown to be as effective, if not more, as anti-depressant medications for alleviating depression.

HOW MUCH EXERCISE IS ENOUGH?

To gain all the benefits that exercise can provide against cancer, you need to be quite active! While moderate activity on a regular basis lowers the risk of cancer, evidence suggests that higher amounts of physical activity may provide even greater reductions in risk. To reduce the risk of breast cancer, you need to walk for thirty to sixty minutes, five days a week.

For colon cancer, vigorous activity may have even greater benefits. Research on colon and prostate cancers has shown that protection is achieved with more intense activities.

Although the optimal intensity, duration, and frequency of physical activity needed to reduce cancer risk are unknown, approaching and exceeding 300 minutes of moderate-intensity activity per week or 150 minutes of vigorous activity per week is likely to provide additional protection against cancer. So instead of walking at a slow pace, try to spend more time on activities and sports such as swimming, walking at a quick pace of around 6 km/hour, jogging, cycling, playing tennis, doing aerobics, and training in martial arts.

Suggestions:

- Exercise reduces cancer risk both directly and indirectly.
- Cancer prevention is stronger as the intensity of the activities gets higher.
- Aim for 300 minutes of moderate-intensity activity per week or 150 minutes of vigorous activity per week.

SUMMARY OF MAIN NUTRITION
RELATED ACTIONS TO LOWER
YOUR CANCER RISK

- Aim to reach and maintain a healthy weight by making positive and permanent changes in your diet and increasing exercise

- Check your vitamin D levels as part of your routine blood tests. Aim to keep your vitamin D levels at least between 40 and 60 ng/ml year-round.

- Eat two to three portions of fruit and three to seven portions of vegetables each day.

- Avoid processed foods, sugar, and salt in order to make your diet more alkalizing.

- Ensure optimum antioxidant protection by aiming for an intake of around 6,000 ORAC units a day. Pick at least three options from the following list : ½ teaspoon ground cinnamon, dried oregano or ground turmeric, 1/5 cup blueberries, ½ pear or grapefruit or 1 plum, ½ cup of black currants, berries, raspberries, or strawberries, ½ cup cherries, 1 orange or 1 apple , 4 pieces of dark chocolate (70% cocoa), 7 walnut halves, 8 pecan halves, ½ cup cooked lentils or 1 cup cooked kidney beans, 1/3 medium avocado, ½ cup red cabbage, 2 cups broccoli, 1 medium artichoke or 8 asparagus spears.

- Eat four to five servings of fresh, dried or frozen berries per week, including grapes.

- Eat pomegranates daily when they are in season. Drink a glass of pure unsweetened pomegranate juice one to two times per week for the rest of the year.

- Include cruciferous vegetables in your diet most days of the week.

- Choose plums, peaches, and nectarines as your snack between meals when they are in season. If possible get organic to avoid the heavy contamination with pesticides.

- Try to eat medicinal mushrooms twice a week. Choose shiitake, maitake, enokitake, cremini, Portobello, or oyster (or pleurotus), as they are richer in the immune-enhancing compounds.

- Add turmeric to your meals as a flavoring in rice, salad dressings, soups, and other dishes. Add a pinch of black pepper to these dishes to aid turmeric absorption by the body.

- Include green tea in your diet as often as possible. Aim to have two to three cups of green tea per day.

- Add garlic to your meals as often as possible, together with onions, and leeks.

- Use herbs and spices extensively in your cooking, as they do have a strong anticancer potential.

- Add seaweed in your diet as often as possible.

- Drink a glass of fresh pineapple juice regularly and include it in your smoothies.

- Eat 120 to 150 grams of fatty fish two to three times a week. If possible, choose meat and dairy products from grass-fed animals, as they contain EPA and DHA. Avoid omega-6-rich oils to maintain a good balance of omega-3 to omega-6.

- Use grated flaxseeds in your muesli, salads, yogurt, and other recipes, as grinding enables the absorption of the beneficial omega-3 fatty acids.

- Make extra-virgin olive oil the main oil you use in your salads and meals. Use 3-4 tablespoons per day.

- Eat one or two Brazil nuts daily.

- Enjoy dark chocolate as a snack two to three times a week. A good portion is around 20 grams.

- To ensure a good intake of dietary fiber choose a whole, plant-based diet and eat legumes (such as beans, chickpeas, peas, and lentils) two to three times per week. Make vegetables the largest part of your meals and aim to have a couple of vegetarian meals each week.

- Have a probiotic rich food, drink or supplement daily. Good options include kefir, plain sheep's yogurt made with lactic acid bacteria or fermented vegetables such as sauerkraut.

- Limit the amount of sugar in the diet by switching to a diet of whole, unprocessed foods. Avoid simple sugars such as sweetened drinks, desserts, honey, molasses, juices, and the like. Limit desserts to special occasions.

- If you are overweight, losing weight will help in better blood sugar control. Test your fasting blood sugar and HβA1c levels often in order to detect at the earliest stages any metabolic effects leading to type II diabetes.

- Aim not to exceed 300 - 500 grams (11 - 18 ounces) of cooked red meat per week and try to avoid processed meat altogether.

- Make sure you keep your meat and fish moist while cooking in order to minimize the heterocyclic amines produced. Prefer stewing, boiling, steaming or poaching when cooking your protein foods.

- Marinate meat, chicken and other white meat or fish in olive oil and herbs to significantly reduce the production of the toxic heterocyclic amines.

- Avoid overcooking when baking, frying, grilling, roasting, or toasting carbohydrate-rich foods by keeping the duration of cooking as short as possible.

- Avoid potato chips and French fries, as they have been found to have the highest amounts of the carcinogenic chemical acrylamide.

- Avoid foods that are heavily salted, smoked, or pickled. Choose a diet consisting of mainly unprocessed foods and avoid ready-made meals or snacks. Replace salt in your meals with herbs.

- Avoid trans fats by avoiding processed and fried foods. Check the labels of the products you buy. Avoid products with hydrogenated or partially hydrogenated oils in their ingredients list, mostly cakes, crackers, biscuits, pie crusts, and some cereal bars.

- Avoid processed food products with additives and choose foods in their original form (i.e., pure cheese instead of processed cheese spreads).

- Check the labels of the products you buy and avoid products with carrageenan, especially if you have digestive issues such as abdominal pain, intestinal bloating, spastic colon, irritable bowel syndrome, ulcerative colitis, Crohn's disease or colon cancer.

- Apply a water filter system to your drinking water.

- Reduce arsenic in your rice by using plenty of water when cooking and by washing the rice in plenty of water before cooking.

- Avoid home fragrances. Replace them with natural essential oils.

- Try to stay informed about environmental and dietary carcinogens such as pesticides, dioxins, and minimize your exposure to them.

- Reducing your exposure to BPA by avoiding plastic food and drink containers. Use glass, pyrex, porcelain, ceramic, or stainless steel containers for hot foods and liquids instead.

- Never heat your food in plastic.

- Avoid using canned foods, since most cans are lined with BPA-containing resin. Examples are tinned fish, such as tuna and sardines, tinned soups, and tined fruits and vegetables.

- Avoid household cleaners and cosmetics with 'fragrance' on the label.

- Avoid nonstick cookware.

- Minimize exposure to pesticides by washing your fruits and vegetables in a bowl of water with two to three tablespoons of vinegar. Let them soak in it for about ten minutes. If possible, choose organically grown fruits and vegetables and get informed on the yearly Dirty Dozen list.

- Keep alcohol intake at very low levels.

- Ensure optimum detoxification of the body by having a high fiber diet with a lot of fruit and vegetables, exercising regularly and drinking a lot of clean water.

- Consider supplementing with milk thistle for a few weeks, a few times per year, to enable the best functioning of your liver. Add foods and herbs with detoxing powers in your diet as often as possible, such as broccoli, beetroots, artichokes, garlic, lemon and coriander.

- Follow a supervised detox or cleansing program once or twice per year to ensure optimal elimination of toxins and for giving a helping hand to your toxin elimination organs.

- Aim for 300 minutes of moderate-intensity activity per week or 150 minutes of vigorous activity per week.

YOUR PERSONAL ROAD TO CANCER PREVENTION

The purpose of this book was to educate you on the multiple ways by which diet can affect cancer risk and to inspire you to make the necessary changes in your diet to help in the prevention of cancer. Reading the book was the first step towards a healthier lifestyle. If you have not already done so, now is the time for you to implement what you have learned and to create new eating habits for you and your loved ones.

ANTICANCER – NUTRITIONAL SELF ASSESSMENT

In order to benefit the most from reading this book, we have created an online interactive tool that assesses your personal nutritional factors that affect cancer risk.

This is a more detailed assessment than the one you had access to at the beginning of the book. The Anticancer Nutritional Self Assessment has been created in order to provide you with personalized tips and to help you concentrate on the specific actions you can take to improve your nutrition and optimize your diet's anticancer potential. To find the questionnaire follow the link below:

www.mynutrilosophy.com/anticancer/step-2-assessment

Simply visit the above link and answer the questions of the self assessment. After completing the assessment you will receive your personal 'Nutritional Factors Profile for Cancer Prevention' which will outline the recommended nutrition and lifestyle changes specific to you that will make the biggest impact on your cancer risk.

Once you obtain your personal 'Nutritional Factors Profile for Cancer Prevention' you can save or print it out for future reference.

You may want to come back in the future and complete a new Nutritional Self Assessment, as your habits and lifestyle will change over time. This will ensure that you refresh the important steps you need to be doing regularly in order to reduce your lifetime cancer risk.

BIBLIOGRAPHY

PART A
Introduction to Cancer

Chapter 1: What Is Cancer?

1. What is Cancer? National Cancer Institute, http://www.cancer.gov/about-cancer/what-is-cancer
2. Pine, Sharon R., and Wenyu Liu. "Asymmetric cell division and template DNA co-segregation in cancer stem cells." *Frontiers in oncology* 4 (2014).
3. Worldwide cancer incidence statistics, Cancer Research UK, http://www.cancerresearchuk.org/health-professional/cancer-statistics/worldwide-cancer/incidence#JvY8K2eYAsY-8WUD8.99
4. Ahmad, A. S., N. Ormiston-Smith, and P. D. Sasieni. "Trends in the lifetime risk of developing cancer in Great Britain: comparison of risk for those born from 1930 to 1960." *British journal of cancer* 112, no. 5 (2015): 943-947.

Chapter 2: Is It All in the Genes or Do We Have the Chance to React?

1. Family Cancer Syndromes, American Cancer Society, http://www.cancer.org/cancer/cancercauses/geneticsandcancer/heredity-and-cancer
2. Anand, Preetha, Ajaikumar B. Kunnumakara, Chitra Sundaram, Kuzhuvelil B. Harikumar, Sheeja T. Tharakan, Oiki S. Lai, Bokyung Sung, and Bharat B. Aggarwal. "Cancer is a preventa-

ble disease that requires major lifestyle changes." *Pharmaceutical research* 25, no. 9 (2008): 2097-2116.

3. Supic, Gordana, Maja Jagodic, and Zvonko Magic. "Epigenetics: a new link between nutrition and cancer." *Nutrition and cancer* 65, no. 6 (2013): 781-792.

4. Ghadirian, Parviz, Steven Narod, Eve Fafard, Myriam Costa, André Robidoux, and André Nkondjock. "Breast cancer risk in relation to the joint effect of BRCA mutations and diet diversity." *Breast cancer research and treatment* 117, no. 2 (2009): 417-422.

5. Cancer Prevention, World Health Organization, http://www.who.int/cancer/prevention/en/

6. Cancer linked with poor nutrition, World Health Organization, Regional office for Europe, http://www.euro.who.int/en/health-topics/noncommunicable-diseases/cancer/news/news/2011/02/cancer-linked-with-poor-nutrition

7. Reduce your cancer risk, American Institute for Cancer Research, http://www.aicr.org/reduce-your-cancer-risk/

8. Cancer prevention: Putting it together, American Institute for Cancer Research, http://www.aicr.org/reduce-your-cancer-risk/cancer-prevention

9. Cancer Preventability, American Institute for Cancer Research, http://www.aicr.org/learn-more-about-cancer/infographics-cancer-preventability.html

PART B
Weight–Cancer Link

Chapter 3: Reduce Cancer Risk by Maintaining a Healthy Weight

1. Ligibel, Jennifer A., Catherine M. Alfano, Kerry S. Courneya, Wendy Demark-Wahnefried, Robert A. Burger, Rowan T. Chle-

bowski, Carol J. Fabian et al. "American Society of Clinical On-cology position statement on obesity and cancer." *Journal of clinical oncology* 32, no. 31 (2014): 3568-3574.

2. Cancer linked with poor nutrition, World Health Organiza-tion, http://www.euro.who.int/en/health-topics/noncommu-nicable-diseases/cancer/news/news/2011/02/cancer-linked-with-poor-nutrition

3. Basen-Engquist, Karen, and Maria Chang. "Obesity and can-cer risk: recent review and evidence." *Current oncology re-ports* 13, no. 1 (2011): 71-76.

4. Battle of the bulge tips the scales on cancer war, University of Colorado Cancer Center, http://www.coloradocancerblogs.org/battle-of-the-bulge-tips-the-scales-on-cancer-war/

5. The Weight-Cancer Link, American Institute for Cancer Re-search, http://www.aicr.org/reduce-your-cancer-risk/weight/reduce_weight_cancer_link.html

6. World Cancer Research Fund / American Institute for Cancer Research. Food, Nutrition, Physical Activity, and the Prevention of Cancer: a Global Perspective. Washington DC: AICR, 2007

Chapter 4: The Importance of Weight after a Cancer Diagnosis

1. Protani, Melinda, Michael Coory, and Jennifer H. Martin. "Effect of obesity on survival of women with breast cancer: systematic review and meta-analysis."*Breast cancer research and treatment* 123, no. 3 (2010): 627-635.

2. Dowsett, Mitch, Jack Cuzick, Jim Ingle, Alan Coates, John Forbes, Judith Bliss, Marc Buyse et al. "Meta-analysis of breast cancer outcomes in adjuvant trials of aromatase in-hibitors versus tamoxifen." *Journal of Clinical Oncology* 28, no. 3 (2010): 509-518.

3. McCarroll, M. L., S. Armbruster, H. E. Frasure, M. D. Gothard, K. M. Gil, M. B. Kavanagh, S. Waggoner, and V. E. Von Gruenigen. "Self-efficacy, quality of life, and weight loss in overweight/obese endometrial cancer survivors (SUCCEED): a randomized controlled trial." *Gynecologic oncology* 132, no. 2 (2014): 397-402.
4. Overweight and obese cancer survivors benefit from weight loss program, Cure, http://www.curetoday.com/articles/overweight-and-obese-cancer-survivors-benefit-from-weight-loss-program
5. Phillips, Siobhan M., and Edward McAuley. "Associations between self-reported post-diagnosis physical activity changes, body weight changes, and psychosocial well-being in breast cancer survivors." *Supportive Care in Cancer* 23, no. 1 (2015): 159-167.
6. Weight gain during cancer treatment, American Cancer Society, http://blogs.cancer.org/expertvoices/2012/07/05/weight-gain-during-cancer-treatment/?_ga=1.200702766.10328849 86.1421620301

PART C
Vitamin D

Chapter 5: Vitamin D and Cancer: A New Role for Vitamin D

1. Overview how much vitamin D, http://www.vitamindwiki.com/Overview+How+Much +vitamin+D
2. Holick, Michael F. "Sunlight and vitamin D for bone health and prevention of autoimmune diseases, cancers, and cardiovascular disease." *The American journal of clinical nutrition* 80, no. 6 (2004): 1678S-1688S.
3. Gorham, Edward D., Cedric F. Garland, Frank C. Garland, William B. Grant, Sharif B. Mohr, Martin Lipkin, Harold L.

Newmark, Edward Giovannucci, Melissa Wei, and Michael F. Holick. "Vitamin D and prevention of colorectal cancer." *The Journal of steroid biochemistry and molecular biology* 97, no. 1 (2005): 179-194.

4. http://www.grassrootshealth.net/index.php/press-20100823

5. Cheung, Florence SG, Frank J. Lovicu, and Juergen KV Reichardt. "Current progress in using vitamin D and its analogs for cancer prevention and treatment." *Expert review of anticancer therapy* 12, no. 6 (2012): 811-837.

6. Krishnan, Aruna V., and David Feldman. "Mechanisms of the anti-cancer and anti-inflammatory actions of vitamin D." *Annual review of pharmacology and toxicology* 51 (2011): 311-336.

7. Moreno, Jacqueline, Aruna V. Krishnan, Donna M. Peehl, and David Feldman. "Mechanisms of vitamin D-mediated growth inhibition in prostate cancer cells: inhibition of the prostaglandin pathway." *Anticancer research* 26, no. 4A (2006): 2525-2530.

8. Garland, Cedric F, Frank C Garland, Eddie Ko Shaw, George W Comstock, Knud J Helsing, and Edward D Gorham. "Serum 25-hydroxyvitamin D and colon cancer: eight-year prospective study." *The Lancet* 334, no. 8673 (1989): 1176-1178.

9. Rose, April AN, Christine Elser, Marguerite Ennis, and Pamela J. Goodwin. "Blood levels of vitamin D and early stage breast cancer prognosis: a systematic review and meta-analysis." *Breast cancer research and treatment* 141, no. 3 (2013): 331-339.

10. Goodwin, Pamela J., Marguerite Ennis, Kathleen I. Pritchard, Jarley Koo, and Nicky Hood. "Prognostic effects of 25-hydroxyvitamin D levels in early breast cancer." *Journal of Clinical Oncology* 27, no. 23 (2009): 3757-3763.

11. Garland, Cedric F., Edward D. Gorham, Sharif B. Mohr, and Frank C. Garland. "Vitamin D for cancer prevention: global perspective." *Annals of epidemiology* 19, no. 7 (2009): 468-483.

12. Baek, Sungmin, Young-Suk Lee, Hye-Eun Shim, Sik Yoon, Sun-Yong Baek, Bong-Seon Kim, and Sae-Ock Oh. "Vitamin D3 regulates cell viability in gastric cancer and cholangiocarcinoma." *Anatomy & cell biology* 44, no. 3 (2011): 204-209.

Chapter 6: Optimize Your Vitamin D levels

1. Garland, Cedric F., Edward D. Gorham, Sharif B. Mohr, and Frank C. Garland. "Vitamin D for cancer prevention: global perspective." *Annals of epidemiology* 19, no. 7 (2009): 468-483.
2. Garland, Cedric F., Edward D. Gorham, Sharif B. Mohr, and Frank C. Garland. "Vitamin D for cancer prevention: global perspective." *Annals of epidemiology* 19, no. 7 (2009): 468-483.
3. Vitamin D Council, www.vitamindouncil.org
4. https://www.vitamindcouncil.org/about-vitamin-d/how-do-i-get-the-vitamin-d-my-body-needs
5. Dr. Kate Rheaume-Bleue, "Vitamin K2 and the Calcium Paradox: How a Little-Known Vitamin Could Save Your Life"

PART D
Increase Consumption of the Foods that Fight Cancer

Chapter 7: Cancer Prevention through Food

1. Cancer linked with poor nutrition, World Health Organization,
2. "Foods to Fight Cancer", by Professor Richard Beliveau and Dr. Denis Gingras, 2007, ISBN 978-1-4053-1915-7, DK

Chapter 8: Fruits and Vegetables

1. Promoting fruit and vegetable consumption around the world, World Health Organization, http://www.who.int/dietphysicalactivity/fruit/en/\
2. Fruit and Vegetables, IARC Handbooks of Cancer Prevention, WHO, Volume 8, 2003, ISBN 92 832 3008 6

3. Reccomendations for cancer prevention, American Institute for Cancer Research: http://www.aicr.org/reduce-your-cancer-risk/recommendations-for-cancer-prevention/recommendations_04_plant_based.html

4. Cancer and Acid-Base Balance: Busting the Myth, American Institute for Cancer Research, http://preventcancer.aicr.org/site/News2?id=13441

5. A list of acid / alkaline forming foods, http://www.rense.com/1.mpicons/acidalka.htm

6. Schwalfenberg, Gerry K. "The alkaline diet: is there evidence that an alkaline pH diet benefits health?." *Journal of Environmental and Public Health* 2012 (2011).

Chapter 9: Antioxidants, Free Radicals, and Cancer

1. Fang, Yun-Zhong, Sheng Yang, and Guoyao Wu. "Free radicals, antioxidants, and nutrition." *Nutrition* 18, no. 10 (2002): 872-879.

2. Patrick Holford "Say No to Cancer", updated edition 2010, ISBN 978-0-7499-5411-6.

3. Stoner, Gary David, Li-Shu Wang, and Bruce Cordell Casto. "Laboratory and clinical studies of cancer chemoprevention by antioxidants in berries."*Carcinogenesis* 29, no. 9 (2008): 1665-1674.

4. Stoner, Gary D. "Foodstuffs for preventing cancer: the preclinical and clinical development of berries." *Cancer Prevention Research* 2, no. 3 (2009): 187-194.

5. Stoner, Gary D., Li-Shu Wang, Nancy Zikri, Tong Chen, Stephen S. Hecht, Chuanshu Huang, Christine Sardo, and John F. Lechner. "Cancer prevention with freeze-dried berries and berry components." In *Seminars in cancer biology*, vol. 17, no. 5, pp. 403-410. Academic Press, 2007.

6. Stoner, Gary D. "Foodstuffs for preventing cancer: the preclinical and clinical development of berries." *Cancer Prevention Research* 2, no. 3 (2009): 187-194.

7. Berries seem to burst with cancer prevention, American Institute for Cancer Research, http://www.aicr.org/publications/newsletter/2013-spring-119/berries-seem-to-burst-with-cancer-prevention.html

8. Mertens-Talcott, Susanne U., Joon-Hee Lee, Susan S. Percival, and Stephen T. Talcott. "Induction of cell death in Caco-2 human colon carcinoma cells by ellagic acid rich fractions from muscadine grapes (Vitis rotundifolia)."*Journal of agricultural and food chemistry* 54, no. 15 (2006): 5336-5343.

9. Narayanan, Bhagavathi A., and Gian G. Re. "IGF-II down regulation associated cell cycle arrest in colon cancer cells exposed to phenolic antioxidant ellagic acid." *Anticancer research* 21, no. 1A (2000): 359-364.

10. Kresty, Laura A., Mark A. Morse, Charlotte Morgan, Peter S. Carlton, Jerry Lu, Ashok Gupta, Michelle Blackwood, and Gary D. Stoner. "Chemoprevention of esophageal tumorigenesis by dietary administration of lyophilized black raspberries." *Cancer Research* 61, no. 16 (2001): 6112-6119.

11. Zhang, Zhiping, Xiaoming Liu, Tao Wu, Junhong Liu, Xu Zhang, Xueyun Yang, Michael J. Goodheart, John F. Engelhardt, and Yujiong Wang. "Selective suppression of cervical cancer Hela cells by 2-O-β-d-glucopyranosyl-l-ascorbic acid isolated from the fruit of Lycium barbarum L."*Cell biology and toxicology* 27, no. 2 (2011): 107-121.

12. Cassileth, Barrie. "Lycium (Lycium barbarum)." *Oncology (Williston Park, NY)*24, no. 14 (2010): 1353-1353.

13. Amagase, Harunobu, Buxiang Sun, and Carmia Borek. "Lycium barbarum (goji) juice improves in vivo antioxidant bio-

markers in serum of healthy adults." *Nutrition Research* 29, no. 1 (2009): 19-25.

14. Tang, Wai-Man, Enoch Chan, Ching-Yee Kwok, Yee-Ki Lee, Jian-Hong Wu, Chun-Wai Wan, Robbie Yat-Kan Chan, Peter Hoi-Fu Yu, and Shun-Wan Chan. "A review of the anticancer and immunomodulatory effects of Lycium barbarum fruit." *Inflammopharmacology* 20, no. 6 (2012): 307-314.

15. Zhu, You-Ping. *Chinese materia medica: chemistry, pharmacology and applications.* CRC Press, 1998.

16. Lu, C. X., and B. Q. Cheng. "[Radiosensitizing effects of Lycium barbarum polysaccharide for Lewis lung cancer]." *Zhong xi yi jie he za zhi= Chinese journal of modern developments in traditional medicine/Zhongguo Zhong xi yi jie he yan jiu hui (chou), Zhong yi yan jiu yuan, zhu ban* 11, no. 10 (1991): 611-2.

17. Cao, G. W., W. G. Yang, and Ping Du. "[Observation of the effects of LAK/IL-2 therapy combining with Lycium barbarum polysaccharides in the treatment of 75 cancer patients]." *Zhonghua zhong liu za zhi [Chinese journal of oncology]* 16, no. 6 (1994): 428-431.

18. Li, Go, Daniel W. Sepkovic, H. Leon Bradlow, Nitin T. Telang, and George YC Wong. "Lycium barbarum inhibits growth of estrogen receptor positive human breast cancer cells by favorably altering estradiol metabolism." *Nutrition and cancer* 61, no. 3 (2009): 408-414.

Chapter 10: The Most Anticancer Fruits and Vegetables

1. Schaefer, Brian A., Catherine Dooner, M. Danny Burke, and Gerard A. Potter. "Nutrition and cancer: further case studies involving Salvestrol."*Journal of Orthomolecular Medicine* 25, no. 1 (2010): 17.

2. Foods that fight cancer, Grapes and grape juice, American Institute for Cancer Research, http://www.aicr.org/foods-that-fight-cancer/foodsthatfightcancer_grapes_and_grape_juice.html

3. Csiszar, Anna. "Anti-inflammatory effects of resveratrol: possible role in prevention of age-related cardiovascular disease." *Annals of the New York Academy of Sciences* 1215, no. 1 (2011): 117-122.

4. Fernández, Agustín F., and Mario F. Fraga. "The effects of the dietary polyphenol resveratrol on human healthy aging and lifespan." *Epigenetics* 6, no. 7 (2011): 870-874.

5. Kim, InYoung, and Yu-Ying He. "Targeting the AMP-activated protein kinase for cancer prevention and therapy." *Frontiers in oncology* 3 (2013): 175.

6. Zhu, Hai-Liang. "Resveratrol and its analogues: promising antitumor agents."*Anti-Cancer Agents in Medicinal Chemistry (Formerly Current Medicinal Chemistry-Anti-Cancer Agents)* 11, no. 5 (2011): 479-490.

7. Athar, Mohammad, Jung Ho Back, Xiuwei Tang, Kwang Ho Kim, Levy Kopelovich, David R. Bickers, and Arianna L. Kim. "Resveratrol: a review of preclinical studies for human cancer prevention." *Toxicology and applied pharmacology* 224, no. 3 (2007): 274-283.

8. Longtin, Robert. "The pomegranate: nature's power fruit?." *Journal of the National Cancer Institute* 95, no. 5 (2003): 346-348.

9. Adhami, Vaqar Mustafa, Naghma Khan, and Hasan Mukhtar. "Cancer chemoprevention by pomegranate: laboratory and clinical evidence." *Nutrition and cancer* 61, no. 6 (2009): 811-815.

10. Gil, Maria I., Francisco A. Tomás-Barberán, Betty Hess-Pierce, Deirdre M. Holcroft, and Adel A. Kader. "Antioxidant activity of pomegranate juice and its relationship with phenolic com-

position and processing." *Journal of Agricultural and Food chemistry* 48, no. 10 (2000): 4581-4589.

11. Noda, Yasuko, Takao Kaneyuki, Akitane Mori, and Lester Packer. "Antioxidant activities of pomegranate fruit extract and its anthocyanidins: delphinidin, cyanidin, and pelargonidin." *Journal of Agricultural and Food Chemistry* 50, no. 1 (2002): 166-171.

12. Schubert, Shay Yehoshua, Ephraim Philip Lansky, and Ishak Neeman. "Antioxidant and eicosanoid enzyme inhibition properties of pomegranate seed oil and fermented juice flavonoids." *Journal of ethnopharmacology* 66, no. 1 (1999): 11-17.

13. Lansky, Ephraim P., Wenguo Jiang, Huanbiao Mo, Lou Bravo, Paul Froom, Weiping Yu, Neil M. Harris, Ishak Neeman, and Moray J. Campbell. "Possible synergistic prostate cancer suppression by anatomically discrete pomegranate fractions." *Investigational new drugs* 23, no. 1 (2005): 11-20.

14. Adhami, Vaqar Mustafa, Naghma Khan, and Hasan Mukhtar. "Cancer chemoprevention by pomegranate: laboratory and clinical evidence." *Nutrition and cancer* 61, no. 6 (2009): 811-815.

15. Pantuck, Allan J., John T. Leppert, Nazy Zomorodian, William Aronson, Jenny Hong, R. James Barnard, Navindra Seeram et al. "Phase II study of pomegranate juice for men with rising prostate-specific antigen following surgery or radiation for prostate cancer." *Clinical Cancer Research* 12, no. 13 (2006): 4018-4026.

16. Pantuck, Allan J., John T. Leppert, Nazy Zomorodian, William Aronson, Jenny Hong, R. James Barnard, Navindra Seeram et al. "Phase II study of pomegranate juice for men with rising prostate-specific antigen following surgery or radiation for prostate cancer." *Clinical Cancer Research* 12, no. 13 (2006): 4018-4026.

17. Paller, C. J., X. Ye, P. J. Wozniak, B. K. Gillespie, P. R. Sieber, R. H. Greengold, B. R. Stockton et al. "A randomized phase II study of pomegranate extract for men with rising PSA following initial therapy for localized prostate cancer." *Prostate cancer and prostatic diseases* 16, no. 1 (2013): 50-55.

18. Stenner-Liewen, Frank, Heike Liewen, Richard Cathomas, Christoph Renner, Ulf Petrausch, Tullio Sulser, Katharina Spanaus et al. "Daily pomegranate intake has no impact on PSA levels in patients with advanced prostate cancer—results of a phase IIb randomized controlled trial." *J Cancer* 4, no. 7 (2013): 597-605.

19. Beecher, C. Wf. "Cancer preventive properties of varieties of Brassica oleracea: a review." *The American journal of clinical nutrition* 59, no. 5 (1994): 1166S-1170S

20. .Professor Richard Beliveau and Dr. Denis Gingras. Foods to fight cancer. Essential foods to help prevent cancer. Published 2017, ISBN 978-1-4053-1915-7

21. Patrick Holford "Say No to Cancer", updated edition 2010, ISBN 978-0-7499-5411-6.

22. International Agency for Research on Cancer. *Cruciferous vegetables, isothiocyanates and indoles.* IARC, 2004.

23. Feasting with Cruciferous for Cancer Prevention, American Institute for Cancer Research, http://preventcancer.aicr.org/site/News2?id=19792

24. Foods that fight cancer, Broccoli, American Institute for Cancer Research, http://www.aicr.org/foods-that-fight-cancer/broccoli-cruciferous.html

25. Noratto, Giuliana, Weston Porter, David Byrne, and Luis Cisneros-Zevallos. "Identifying peach and plum polyphenols with chemopreventive potential against estrogen-independent breast cancer cells." *Journal of agricultural and food chemistry* 57, no. 12 (2009): 5219-5226.

26. Ikekawa, Tetsuro, Nobuaki Uehara, Yuko Maeda, Miyako Na-
    kanishi, and Fumiko Fukuoka. "Antitumor activity of aqueous
    extracts of edible mushrooms." *Cancer Research* 29, no. 3
    (1969): 734-735.

27. Li, Jiaoyuan, Li Zou, Wei Chen, Beibei Zhu, Na Shen, Juntao
    Ke, Jiao Lou, Ranran Song, Rong Zhong, and Xiaoping Miao.
    "Dietary mushroom intake may reduce the risk of breast can-
    cer: evidence from a meta-analysis of observational studies."
    PloS one 9, no. 4 (2014): e93437.

28. Shin, Aesun, Jeongseon Kim, Sun-Young Lim, Gaeul Kim, Mi-
    Kyung Sung, Eun-Sook Lee, and Jungsil Ro. "Dietary mush-
    room intake and the risk of breast cancer based on hormone re-
    ceptor status." *Nutrition and cancer* 62, no. 4 (2010): 476-483.

29. Torisu, Motomichi, Yoshihiko Hayashi, Toshiyuki Ishimitsu,
    Takeshi Fujimura, Kazunori Iwasaki, Mitsuo Katano, Hiro-
    shi Yamamoto et al. "Significant prolongation of disease-free
    period gained by oral polysaccharide K (PSK) administration
    after curative surgical operation of colorectal cancer." *Cancer
    Immunology, Immunotherapy* 31, no. 5 (1990): 261-268.

30. Sengupta, Archana, Samit Ghosh, and Shamee Bhattacharjee.
    "Allium vegetables in cancer prevention: an overview." *Asian
    Pacific Journal of Cancer Prevention* 5, no. 3 (2004): 237-245.

31. HERMAN-ANTOSIEWICZ, Anna, Anna A. Powolny, and
    Shivendra V. Singh. "Molecular targets of cancer chemopre-
    vention by garlic-derived organosulfides1." *Acta pharmaco-
    logica Sinica* 28, no. 9 (2007): 1355-1364.

32. Moussavou, Ghislain, Dong Hoon Kwak, Brice Wilfried Obiang-
    Obonou, Cyr Abel Ogandaga Maranguy, Sylvatrie-Danne Din-
    zouna-Boutamba, Dae Hoon Lee, Ordelia Gwenaelle Manvou-
    dou Pissibanganga, Kisung Ko, Jae In Seo, and Young Kug
    Choo. "Anticancer effects of different seaweeds on human

colon and breast cancers." *Marine drugs* 12, no. 9 (2014): 4898-4911.

33. Cancer Treatment Centers of America: "Fucoidan may help fight cancer but research is still early", http://www.cancer-center.com/discussions/blog/fucoidan-may-help-fight-cancer-but-research-is-still-early/

34. Riby, Jacques E., Lucia Conde, Xiangqin Cui, Jianqing Zhang, and Christine F. Skibola. "Mechanisms of anti-tumurogenic activity of the brown seaweed, F. vesiculosus." *Cancer Research* 74, no. 19 Supplement (2014): 5496-5496.

Chapter 11: Cancer Prevention through Herbs and Spices

1. J.Ferlay et al. WHO International Agency for Research on Cancer (IARC), IARC Cancer Epidemiology Database.Globocan 2000. Cancer Incidence, mortality and prevalence worldwide (Lyon, France: IARC Press; 2000).

2. Goel, Ajay, and Bharat B. Aggarwal. "Curcumin, the golden spice from Indian saffron, is a chemosensitizer and radiosensitizer for tumors and chemoprotector and radioprotector for normal organs." *Nutrition and cancer* 62, no. 7 (2010): 919-930.

3. Goel, Ajay, and Bharat B. Aggarwal. "Curcumin, the golden spice from Indian saffron, is a chemosensitizer and radiosensitizer for tumors and chemoprotector and radioprotector for normal organs." *Nutrition and cancer* 62, no. 7 (2010): 919-930.

4. The Benefits of Curcumin in Cancer Treatment, http://articles.mercola.com/sites/articles/archive/2014/03/02/curcumin-benefits.aspx, accessed at 21/1/2015

5. Ravindran, Jayaraj, Sahdeo Prasad, and Bharat B. Aggarwal. "Curcumin and cancer cells: how many ways can curry kill tumor cells selectively?." *The AAPS journal* 11, no. 3 (2009): 495-510.

6. Gao, Xiaohua, Dorrah Deeb, Hao Jiang, Yong B. Liu, Scott A. Dulchavsky, and Subhash C. Gautam. "Curcumin differentially sensitizes malignant glioma cells to TRAIL/Apo2L-mediated apoptosis through activation of procaspases and release of cytochrome c from mitochondria." *Journal of experimental therapeutics & oncology* 5, no. 1 (2005).

7. Goel, Ajay, and Bharat B. Aggarwal. "Curcumin, the golden spice from Indian saffron, is a chemosensitizer and radiosensitizer for tumors and chemoprotector and radioprotector for normal organs." *Nutrition and cancer* 62, no. 7 (2010): 919-930.

8. Dr David Servan-Schreiber, Anti-Cancer : A new Way of life, Penguin Books, ISBN: 978-0-718-15684-8

9. Yuan, Jian-Min, Canlan Sun, and Lesley M. Butler. "Tea and cancer prevention: epidemiological studies." *Pharmacological research* 64, no. 2 (2011): 123-135.

10. Yang, Chung S., Xin Wang, Gang Lu, and Sonia C. Picinich. "Cancer prevention by tea: animal studies, molecular mechanisms and human relevance." *Nature Reviews Cancer* 9, no. 6 (2009): 429-439.

11. Ju, Jihyeung, Jungil Hong, Jian-nian Zhou, Zui Pan, Mousumi Bose, Jie Liao, Guang-yu Yang et al. "Inhibition of intestinal tumorigenesis in Apcmin/+ mice by (–)-epigallocatechin-3-gallate, the major catechin in green tea." *Cancer research* 65, no. 22 (2005): 10623-10631.

12. Higdon, Jane V., and Balz Frei. "Tea catechins and polyphenols: health effects, metabolism, and antioxidant functions." (2003): 89-143.

13. Ju, Jihyeung, Gang Lu, Joshua D. Lambert, and Chung S. Yang. "Inhibition of carcinogenesis by tea constituents." In *Seminars in cancer biology*, vol. 17, no. 5, pp. 395-402. Academic Press, 2007.

14. Yang, Chung S., Pius Maliakal, and Xiaofeng Meng. "Inhibition of Carcinogenesis by Tea*." *Annual Review of Pharmacology and Toxicology*42, no. 1 (2002): 25-54.

15. Nechuta, Sarah, Xiao-Ou Shu, Hong-Lan Li, Gong Yang, Bu-Tian Ji, Yong-Bing Xiang, Hui Cai, Wong-Ho Chow, Yu-Tang Gao, and Wei Zheng. "Prospective cohort study of tea consumption and risk of digestive system cancers: results from the Shanghai Women's Health Study." *The American journal of clinical nutrition* 96, no. 5 (2012): 1056-1063.

16. Lu, Qing-Yi, Lifeng Zhang, Jennifer K. Yee, Vay-Liang W. Go, and Wai-Nang Lee. "Metabolic consequences of LDHA inhibition by epigallocatechin gallate and oxamate in MIA PaCa-2 pancreatic cancer cells." *Metabolomics* 11 (2015): 71-80.

17. http://articles.mercola.com/sites/articles/archive/2009/02/10/three-cups-of-tea-a-day-slashes-your-breast-cancer-risk.aspx

18. Exploring How Green Tea May Protect against Cancer, American Institute of Cancer Research, Spring 2014 Newsletter, http://www.aicr.org/publications/newsletter/2014/123-spring/newsletter-exploring-how-green-tea-may-protect-against-cancer.html

19. Islami, Farhad, Akram Pourshams, Dariush Nasrollahzadeh, Farin Kamangar, Saman Fahimi, Ramin Shakeri, Behnoush Abedi-Ardekani et al. "Tea drinking habits and oesophageal cancer in a high risk area in northern Iran: population based case-control study." (2009): b929.

20. http://articles.mercola.com/sites/articles/archive/2009/04/18/Steaming-Hot-Tea-Linked-to-Cancer.aspx

21. Jia, Li. "Why bortezomib cannot go with 'green'?." *Cancer biology & medicine*10, no. 4 (2013): 206-213.

22. Dragland, Steinar, Haruki Senoo, Kenjiro Wake, Kari Holte, and Rune Blomhoff. "Several culinary and medicinal herbs are

important sources of dietary antioxidants." *The Journal of nutrition* 133, no. 5 (2003): 1286-1290.

23. Solowey, Elisha, Michal Lichtenstein, Sarah Sallon, Helena Paavilainen, Elaine Solowey, and Haya Lorberboum-Galski. "Evaluating medicinal plants for anticancer activity." *The Scientific World Journal* 2014 (2014).

24. Huang, Wu-Yang, Yi-Zhong Cai, and Yanbo Zhang. "Natural phenolic compounds from medicinal herbs and dietary plants: potential use for cancer prevention." *Nutrition and cancer* 62, no. 1 (2009): 1-20.

25. Yi, Weiguang, and Hazel Y. Wetzstein. "Anti-tumorigenic activity of five culinary and medicinal herbs grown under greenhouse conditions and their combination effects." *Journal of the Science of Food and Agriculture* 91, no. 10 (2011): 1849-1854.

26. Johnson, Jeremy J. "Carnosol: a promising anti-cancer and anti-inflammatory agent." *Cancer letters* 305, no. 1 (2011): 1-7.

27. Sung, Bokyung, Sahdeo Prasad, Vivek R. Yadav, and Bharat B. Aggarwal. "Cancer cell signaling pathways targeted by spice-derived nutraceuticals."*Nutrition and cancer* 64, no. 2 (2012): 173-197.

Chapter 12: Enzymes in the Fight against Cancer

1. Chobotova, Katya, Ann B. Vernallis, and Fadzilah Adibah Abdul Majid. "Bromelain's activity and potential as an anti-cancer agent: current evidence and perspectives." *Cancer letters* 290, no. 2 (2010): 148-156.

2. Castell, J. V., G. E. R. H. A. R. D. Friedrich, C. S. Kuhn, and GEORG E. Poppe. "Intestinal absorption of undegraded proteins in men: presence of bromelain in plasma after oral intake." *American Journal of Physiology-Gastrointestinal and Liver Physiology* 273, no. 1 (1997): G139-G146.

3. Bhui, Kulpreet, Shilpa Tyagi, Bharti Prakash, and Yogeshwer Shukla. "Pineapple bromelain induces autophagy, facilitating

apoptotic response in mammary carcinoma cells." *Biofactors* 36, no. 6 (2010): 474-482.

4. Hale, Laura P., Maciej Chichlowski, Chau T. Trinh, and Paula K. Greer. "Dietary supplementation with fresh pineapple juice decreases inflammation and colonic neoplasia in IL-10-deficient mice with colitis." *Inflammatory bowel diseases* 16, no. 12 (2010): 2012-2021.

5. Báez, Roxana, Miriam TP Lopes, Carlos E. Salas, and Martha Hernández. "In vivo antitumoral activity of stem pineapple (Ananas comosus) bromelain."*Planta medica* 73, no. 13 (2007): 1377-1383.

6. Pillai, Krishna, Anahid Ehteda, Javid Akhter, Terence C. Chua, and David L. Morris. "Anticancer effect of bromelain with and without cisplatin or 5-FU on malignant peritoneal mesothelioma cells." *Anti-cancer drugs* 25, no. 2 (2014): 150-160.

7. Bromelain, University of Maryland Medical Center, http://umm.edu/health/medical/altmed/supplement/bromelain#ixzz3QCmltJih University of Maryland Medical Center

8. Can Bromelain Ease Your Pain? https://www.verywell.com/bromelain-what-should-you-know-about-it-88318

Chapter 13: The Role of Good Fats in Cancer Prevention

1. Giacosa, Attilio, Roberto Barale, Luigi Bavaresco, Piers Gatenby, Vincenzo Gerbi, Jaak Janssens, Belinda Johnston et al. "Cancer prevention in Europe: the Mediterranean diet as a protective choice." *European Journal of Cancer Prevention* 22, no. 1 (2013): 90-95.

2. Trichopoulou, Antonia, Pagona Lagiou, Hannah Kuper, and Dimitrios Trichopoulos. "Cancer and Mediterranean dietary traditions." *Cancer Epidemiology Biomarkers & Prevention* 9, no. 9 (2000): 869-873.

3. Simopoulos, A. P. "The traditional diet of Greece and cancer." *European Journal of Cancer Prevention* 13, no. 3 (2004): 219-230.

4. Pauwels, Ernest KJ. "The protective effect of the Mediterranean diet: focus on cancer and cardiovascular risk." *Medical principles and practice* 20, no. 2 (2011): 103-111.

5. Myrna Brind Center of Integrative Medicine; The Use of Fatty Acids in Malignancies, July 2006, http://jdc.jefferson.edu/cgi/viewcontent.cgi?article=1003&context=jmbcim

6. Stephenson, James Andrew, Omer Al-Taan, A& al Arshad, Bruno Morgan, Matthew S. Metcalfe, and A. R. Dennison. "The multifaceted effects of omega-3 polyunsaturated Fatty acids on the hallmarks of cancer." *Journal of lipids* 2013 (2013).

7. Kang, Jing X. "The Importance of Omega-6/Omega-3 Fatty Acid Ratio in Cell Function." In *Omega-6/Omega-3 Essential Fatty Acid Ratio: The Scientific Evidence*, vol. 92, pp. 23-36. Karger Publishers, 2004.

8. Pauwels, Ernest KJ. "The protective effect of the Mediterranean diet: focus on cancer and cardiovascular risk." *Medical principles and practice* 20, no. 2 (2011): 103-111.

9. Pauwels, Ernest KJ. "The protective effect of the Mediterranean diet: focus on cancer and cardiovascular risk." *Medical principles and practice* 20, no. 2 (2011): 103-111.

10. Myrna Brind Center of Integrative Medicine; The Use of Fatty Acids in Malignancies, July 2006, http://jdc.jefferson.edu/cgi/viewcontent.cgi?article=1003&context=jmbcim

11. Fernandez, Esteve, Liliane Chatenoud, Carlo La Vecchia, Eva Negri, and Silvia Franceschi. "Fish consumption and cancer risk." *The American journal of clinical nutrition* 70, no. 1 (1999): 85-90

12. Terry, Paul, Alicja Wolk, Harri Vainio, and Elisabete Weiderpass. "Fatty Fish Consumption Lowers the Risk of Endometrial Cancer A Nationwide Case-Control Study in Sweden." *Can-*

*cer Epidemiology Biomarkers & Prevention*11, no. 1 (2002): 143-145.

13. Wu, Shengjun, Bin Feng, Kai Li, Xia Zhu, Shuhui Liang, Xufeng Liu, Shuang Han et al. "Fish consumption and colorectal cancer risk in humans: a systematic review and meta-analysis." *The American journal of medicine* 125, no. 6 (2012): 551-559.

14. Jedrychowski, Wieslaw, Umberto Maugeri, Agnieszka Pac, Elzbieta Sochacka-Tatara, and Aleksander Galas. "Protective effect of fish consumption on colorectal cancer risk." *Annals of Nutrition and Metabolism*53, no. 3-4 (2009): 295-302.

15. Kim, Jeongseon, Sun-Young Lim, Aesun Shin, Mi-Kyung Sung, Jungsil Ro, Han-Sung Kang, Keun Seok Lee, Seok-Won Kim, and Eun-Sook Lee. "Fatty fish and fish omega-3 fatty acid intakes decrease the breast cancer risk: a case-control study." *BMC cancer* 9, no. 1 (2009): 1.

16. Rose, David P. "Dietary fatty acids and cancer." *The American journal of clinical nutrition* 66, no. 4 (1997): 998S-1003S.

17. Augustsson, Katarina, Dominique S. Michaud, Eric B. Rimm, Michael F. Leitzmann, Meir J. Stampfer, Walter C. Willett, and Edward Giovannucci. "A prospective study of intake of fish and marine fatty acids and prostate cancer." *Cancer Epidemiology Biomarkers & Prevention* 12, no. 1 (2003): 64-67.

18. Hamilton, M. Coreen, Ronald A. Hites, Steven J. Schwager, Jeffery A. Foran, Barbara A. Knuth, and David O. Carpenter. "Lipid composition and contaminants in farmed and wild salmon." *Environmental science & technology* 39, no. 22 (2005): 8622-8629.

19. Karapanagiotidis, Ioannis T., Michael V. Bell, David C. Little, Amararatne Yakupitiyage, and Sudip K. Rakshit. "Polyunsaturated fatty acid content of wild and farmed tilapias in Thailand: effect of aquaculture practices and implications for

human nutrition." *Journal of agricultural and food chemistry*54, no. 12 (2006): 4304-4310.

20. Young, Kaolin. "Omega-6 (n-6) and omega-3 (n-3) fatty acids in tilapia and human health: a review." *International journal of food sciences and nutrition*60, no. sup5 (2009): 203-211.

21. Top 10 foods highest in omega 3 fatty acids, HealthAlicious-Ness.com, https://www.healthaliciousness.com/articles/high-omega-3-foods.php

22. Hebeisen, Dorothea F., F. Hoeflin, H. P. Reusch, E. Junker, and B. H. Lauterburg. "Increased concentrations of omega-3 fatty acids in milk and platelet rich plasma of grass-fed cows." *International journal for vitamin and nutrition research. Internationale Zeitschrift fur Vitamin-und Ernahrungsforschung. Journal international de vitaminologie et de nutrition*63, no. 3 (1992): 229-233.

23. Hamilton, M. Coreen, Ronald A. Hites, Steven J. Schwager, Jeffery A. Foran, Barbara A. Knuth, and David O. Carpenter. "Lipid composition and contaminants in farmed and wild salmon." *Environmental science & technology* 39, no. 22 (2005): 8622-8629.

24. Khan, Mohammad Rizwan, Rosa Busquets, Javier Saurina, Santiago Hernández, and Lluís Puignou. "Identification of seafood as an important dietary source of heterocyclic amines by chemometry and chromatography–mass spectrometry." *Chemical research in toxicology* 26, no. 6 (2013): 1014-1022.

25. Daley, Cynthia A., Amber Abbott, Patrick S. Doyle, Glenn A. Nader, and Stephanie Larson. "A review of fatty acid profiles and antioxidant content in grass-fed and grain-fed beef." *Nutrition journal* 9, no. 1 (2010): 1.

26. Deckelbaum, Richard J., and Claudia Torrejon. "The omega-3 fatty acid nutritional landscape: health benefits and sources." *The Journal of nutrition*142, no. 3 (2012): 587S-591S.

27. Williams, Christine M., and Graham Burdge. "Long-chain n–3 PUFA: plant v. marine sources." *Proceedings of the Nutrition Society* 65, no. 01 (2006): 42-50.

28. Top 10 foods highest in omega 3 fatty acids, HealthAliciousNess.com, https://www.healthaliciousness.com/articles/high-omega-3-foods.php

29. Flower, Gillian, Heidi Fritz, Lynda G. Balneaves, Shailendra Verma, Becky Skidmore, Rochelle Fernandes, Deborah Kennedy et al. "Flax and breast cancer: A systematic review." *Integrative cancer therapies* (2013): 1534735413502076.

30. Lowcock, Elizabeth C., Michelle Cotterchio, and Beatrice A. Boucher. "Consumption of flaxseed, a rich source of lignans, is associated with reduced breast cancer risk." *Cancer Causes & Control* 24, no. 4 (2013): 813-816.

31. Chen, Jianmin, P. Mark Stavro, and Lilian U. Thompson. "Dietary flaxseed inhibits human breast cancer growth and metastasis and downregulates expression of insulin-like growth factor and epidermal growth factor receptor."*Nutrition and cancer* 43, no. 2 (2002): 187-192.

32. Psaltopoulou, Theodora, Rena I. Kosti, Dimitrios Haidopoulos, Meletios Dimopoulos, and Demosthenes B. Panagiotakos. "Olive oil intake is inversely related to cancer prevalence: a systematic review and a meta-analysis of 13800 patients and 23340 controls in 19 observational studies." *Lipids in health and disease* 10, no. 1 (2011): 1.

33. Barbaro, Barbara, Gabriele Toietta, Roberta Maggio, Mario Arciello, Mirko Tarocchi, Andrea Galli, and Clara Balsano. "Effects of the olive-derived polyphenol oleuropein on human health." *International journal of molecular sciences* 15, no. 10 (2014): 18508-18524.

34. Owen, R. W., R. Haubner, G. Würtele, W. E. Hull, Bartsh Spiegelhalder, and H. Bartsch. "Olives and olive oil in cancer preven-

tion." *European Journal of Cancer Prevention* 13, no. 4 (2004): 319-326.

35. Owen, R. W., R. Haubner, G. Würtele, W. E. Hull, Bartsh Spiegelhalder, and H. Bartsch. "Olives and olive oil in cancer prevention." *European Journal of Cancer Prevention* 13, no. 4 (2004): 319-326.

36. Barbaro, Barbara, Gabriele Toietta, Roberta Maggio, Mario Arciello, Mirko Tarocchi, Andrea Galli, and Clara Balsano. "Effects of the olive-derived polyphenol oleuropein on human health." *International journal of molecular sciences* 15, no. 10 (2014): 18508-18524.

37. Barbaro, Barbara, Gabriele Toietta, Roberta Maggio, Mario Arciello, Mirko Tarocchi, Andrea Galli, and Clara Balsano. "Effects of the olive-derived polyphenol oleuropein on human health." *International journal of molecular sciences* 15, no. 10 (2014): 18508-18524.

Chapter 14: Why You Need a Brazil Nut a Day

1. Barrett, Caitlyn W., Wei Ning, Xi Chen, Jesse Joshua Smith, Mary K. Washington, Kristina E. Hill, Lori A. Coburn et al. "Tumor suppressor function of the plasma glutathione peroxidase gpx3 in colitis-associated carcinoma."*Cancer research* 73, no. 3 (2013): 1245-1255.

2. Iskusnykh, Igor Y., Tatyana N. Popova, Aleksander A. Agarkov, Miguel ÂA Pinheiro de Carvalho, and Stanislav G. Rjevskiy. "Expression of glutathione peroxidase and glutathione reductase and level of free radical processes under toxic hepatitis in rats." *Journal of toxicology* 2013 (2013).

3. Tinggi, Ujang. "Selenium: its role as antioxidant in human health."*Environmental health and preventive medicine* 13, no. 2 (2008): 102-108.

4. Tinggi, Ujang. "Selenium: its role as antioxidant in human health."*Environmental health and preventive medicine* 13, no. 2 (2008): 102-108.

5. Amaral, André FS, Kenneth P. Cantor, Debra T. Silverman, and Núria Malats. "Selenium and bladder cancer risk: a meta-analysis." *Cancer Epidemiology Biomarkers & Prevention* 19, no. 9 (2010): 2407-2415.

6. Rayman, Margaret P. "Selenium and human health." *The Lancet* 379, no. 9822 (2012): 1256-1268

7. Thomson, Christine D., Alexandra Chisholm, Sarah K. McLachlan, and Jennifer M. Campbell. "Brazil nuts: an effective way to improve selenium status." *The American journal of clinical nutrition* 87, no. 2 (2008): 379-384.

Chapter 15: The Benefits of Dark Chocolate: No More Guilt for Loving Your Chocolate

1. Yao, Hua, Weizheng Xu, Xianglin Shi, and Zhuo Zhang. "Dietary flavonoids as cancer prevention agents." *Journal of Environmental Science and Health, Part C* 29, no. 1 (2011): 1-31.

2. Lee, Ki Won, Young Jun Kim, Hyong Joo Lee, and Chang Yong Lee. "Cocoa has more phenolic phytochemicals and a higher antioxidant capacity than teas and red wine." *Journal of agricultural and food chemistry* 51, no. 25 (2003): 7292-7295.

3. Bayard, Vicente, Fermina Chamorro, Jorge Motta, and Norman K. Hollenberg. "Does flavanol intake influence mortality from nitric oxide-dependent processes? Ischemic heart disease, stroke, diabetes mellitus, and cancer in Panama." *International journal of medical sciences* 4, no. 1 (2007): 53.

4. Haritha, K., L. Kalyani, and A. Lakshmana Rao. "Health Benefits of Dark Chocolate." *Journal of Advanced Drug Delivery* 1, no. 4 (2014): 184-194.

5. Vinson, Joe A., John Proch, Pratima Bose, Sean Muchler, Pamela Taffera, Donna Shuta, Najwa Samman, and Gabriel A. Agbor. "Chocolate is a powerful ex vivo and in vivo antioxidant, an antiatherosclerotic agent in an animal model, and a significant contributor to antioxidants in the European and American Diets." *Journal of agricultural and food chemistry* 54, no. 21 (2006): 8071-8076.

6. Romagnolo, Donato F., and Ornella I. Selmin. "Flavonoids and cancer prevention: a review of the evidence." *Journal of nutrition in gerontology and geriatrics* 31, no. 3 (2012): 206-238.

7. Ramos, Sonia, Luis Goya, and Maria Angeles Martín. "Antioxidative Stress Actions of Cocoa in Colonic Cancer." *Cancer: Oxidative Stress and Dietary Antioxidants* (2014): 211.

8. Roura, Elena, Cristina Andrés-Lacueva, Ramon Estruch, M. Lourdes Mata-Bilbao, Maria Izquierdo-Pulido, Andrew L. Waterhouse, and Rosa M. Lamuela-Raventós. "Milk does not affect the bioavailability of cocoa powder flavonoid in healthy human." *Annals of Nutrition and Metabolism* 51, no. 6 (2007): 493-498.

Chapter 16: Dietary Fiber: Why We Need More

1. Yang, Yang, Long-Gang Zhao, Qi-Jun Wu, Xiao Ma, and Yong-Bing Xiang. "Association between dietary fiber and lower risk of all-cause mortality: a meta-analysis of cohort studies." *American journal of epidemiology* 181, no. 2 (2015): 83-91.

2. Hansen, Louise, Guri Skeie, Rikard Landberg, Eiliv Lund, Richard Palmqvist, Ingegerd Johansson, Lars O. Dragsted et al. "Intake of dietary fiber, especially from cereal foods, is associated with lower incidence of colon cancer in the HELGA cohort." *International Journal of Cancer* 131, no. 2 (2012): 469-478.

3. Schatzkin, Arthur, Traci Mouw, Yikyung Park, Amy F. Subar, Victor Kipnis, Albert Hollenbeck, Michael F. Leitzmann, and Frances E. Thompson. "Dietary fiber and whole-grain consumption in relation to colorectal cancer in the NIH-AARP Diet and Health Study." *The American journal of clinical nutrition* 85, no. 5 (2007): 1353-1360.

4. Schatzkin, Arthur, Yikyung Park, Michael F. Leitzmann, Albert R. Hollenbeck, and Amanda J. Cross. "Prospective study of dietary fiber, whole grain foods, and small intestinal cancer." *Gastroenterology* 135, no. 4 (2008): 1163-1167.

5. Chan, Andrew T., and Edward L. Giovannucci. "Primary prevention of colorectal cancer." *Gastroenterology* 138, no. 6 (2010): 2029-2043.

6. Lam, Tram Kim, Amanda J. Cross, Neal Freedman, Yikyung Park, Albert R. Hollenbeck, Arthur Schatzkin, and Christian Abnet. "Dietary fiber and grain consumption in relation to head and neck cancer in the NIH-AARP Diet and Health Study." *Cancer Causes & Control* 22, no. 10 (2011): 1405-1414.

7. Park, Yikyung, Louise A. Brinton, Amy F. Subar, Albert Hollenbeck, and Arthur Schatzkin. "Dietary fiber intake and risk of breast cancer in postmenopausal women: the National Institutes of Health–AARP Diet and Health Study." *The American journal of clinical nutrition* (2009): ajcn-27758.

8. MA, Mendez, Guillem Pera, Antonio Agudo, H. Bas Bueno-de-Mesquita, Domenico Palli, Heiner Boeing, Fatima Carneiro et al. "Cereal fiber intake may reduce risk of gastric adenocarcinomas: The EPIC-EURGAST study. "*International journal of cancer* 121, no. 7 (2007): 1618-1623.

9. Dahm, Christina C., Ruth H. Keogh, Elizabeth A. Spencer, Darren C. Greenwood, Tim J. Key, Ian S. Fentiman, Martin J. Shipley et al. "Dietary fiber and colorectal cancer risk: a nested

case–control study using food diaries." *Journal of the National Cancer Institute* (2010).

10. Dong, Jia-Yi, Ka He, Peiyu Wang, and Li-Qiang Qin. "Dietary fiber intake and risk of breast cancer: a meta-analysis of prospective cohort studies." *The American journal of clinical nutrition* 94, no. 3 (2011): 900-905.

Chapter 17: The Anticancer Role of the Microbes within Us

1. Microbiota, Wikipedia, http://en.wikipedia.org/wiki/Microbiota
2. Probiotics, Wikipedia, http://en.wikipedia.org/wiki/Probiotic
3. FAO/WHO (2006). Probiotics in Food. Health and Nutritional Properties and Guidelines for Evaluation. Rome: FAO Food and Nutrition.
4. Kahouli, Imen, Catherine Tomaro-Duchesneau, and Satya Prakash. "Probiotics in colorectal cancer (CRC) with emphasis on mechanisms of action and current perspectives." *Journal of medical microbiology* 62, no. 8 (2013): 1107-1123.
5. Kahouli, Imen, Catherine Tomaro-Duchesneau, and Satya Prakash. "Probiotics in colorectal cancer (CRC) with emphasis on mechanisms of action and current perspectives." *Journal of medical microbiology* 62, no. 8 (2013): 1107-1123.
6. Khan, Abdul Arif, Mohsin Khurshid, Shahanavaj Khan, and Aws Alshamsan. "Gut microbiota and probiotics: current status and their role in cancer therapeutics." *Drug Development Research* 74, no. 6 (2013): 365-375.
7. Baldwin*, Cindy, Mathieu Millette*, Daniel Oth†, Marcia T. Ruiz, François-Marie Luquet, and Monique Lacroix. "Probiotic Lactobacillus acidophilus and L. casei mix sensitize colorectal tumoral cells to 5-fluorouracil-induced apoptosis." *Nutrition and cancer* 62, no. 3 (2010): 371-378.

8. Österlund, P., T. Ruotsalainen, R. Korpela, M. Saxelin, A. Ollus, P. Valta, M. Kouri, I. Elomaa, and H. Joensuu. "Lactobacillus supplementation for diarrhoea related to chemotherapy of colorectal cancer: a randomised study."*British Journal of Cancer* 97, no. 8 (2007): 1028-1034.

Chapter 18: Tips on Cooking Methods and Food Combinations for Maximum Protection

1. Cooking for Cancer Prevention, American Institue for Cancer Research, http://www.aicr.org/enews/2013/march-2013/Cooking-for-cancer-prevention.html

2. Jacobs Jr, David R. "Food synergy: the key to balancing the nutrition research effort." *Public Health Reviews* 33, no. 2 (2011): 1.

3. Boileau, Thomas W-M., Zhiming Liao, Sunny Kim, Stanley Lemeshow, John W. Erdman Jr, and Steven K. Clinton. "Prostate carcinogenesis in N-methyl-N-nitrosourea (NMU)-testosterone-treated rats fed tomato powder, lycopene, or energy-restricted diets." *Journal of the National Cancer Institute* 95, no. 21 (2003): 1578-1586.

4. Canene-Adams, Kirstie, Brian L. Lindshield, Shihua Wang, Elizabeth H. Jeffery, Steven K. Clinton, and John W. Erdman. "Combinations of tomato and broccoli enhance antitumor activity in dunning r3327-h prostate adenocarcinomas." *Cancer research* 67, no. 2 (2007): 836-843.

5. Thyagarajan, Anita, Jiashi Zhu, and Daniel Sliva. "Combined effect of green tea and Ganoderma lucidum on invasive behavior of breast cancer cells."*International journal of oncology* 30, no. 4 (2007): 963-970.

6. Zhang, Min, Jian Huang, Xing Xie, and CD'Arcy J. Holman. "Dietary intakes of mushrooms and green tea combine to re-

duce the risk of breast cancer in Chinese women." *International-al journal of cancer* 124, no. 6 (2009): 1404-1408.

7. Pathak, A. K., N. Singh, R. Guleria, S. Bal, and S. Thulkar. "Role of vitamins along with chemotherapy in non-small cell lung cancer 2002 International Conference on Nutrition and Cancer Montevideo." *Uruguay, p. 28a (abs.)*(2002).

8. Food-Drug Synergy and Safety – Google Book, 2005, Lilian U.Thompson, Wendy E.Ward. Taylor & Francis

9. Liu, Rui Hai. "Potential synergy of phytochemicals in cancer prevention: mechanism of action." *The Journal of nutrition* 134, no. 12 (2004): 3479S-3485S.

10. Sak, Katrin. "Chemotherapy and dietary phytochemical agents. "*Chemotherapy research and practice* 2012 (2012).

11. Lamson, Davis W., and Matthew S. Brignall. "Antioxidants and cancer therapy II: quick reference guide." *Alternative medicine review: a journal of clinical therapeutic* 5, no. 2 (2000): 152-163.

12. Sagar, Stephen Mark, and Donald Yance. "Natural Health Products that Inhibit Angiogenesis: Part 1." *Current Oncology* 13, no. 1 (2006).

Chapter 19: The Power to Change Our Genes:
The New Science of Epigenetics

1. Gerhauser, Clarissa. "Cancer chemoprevention and nutri-epigenetics: state of the art and future challenges." In *Natural Products in Cancer Prevention and Therapy*, pp. 73-132. Springer Berlin Heidelberg, 2012.

2. Women's Cancer, Translational Research, UCL EGA Institute for women's health, Research Group Leader: Professor Martin Widschwendter, http://www.instituteforwomenshealth.ucl.ac.uk/womens-cancer/trl

3. Link, Alexander, Francesc Balaguer, and Ajay Goel. "Cancer chemoprevention by dietary polyphenols: promising role for epigenetics."*Biochemical pharmacology* 80, no. 12 (2010): 1771-1792.

4. Supic, Gordana, Maja Jagodic, and Zvonko Magic. "Epigenetics: a new link between nutrition and cancer." *Nutrition and cancer* 65, no. 6 (2013): 781-792.

5. Lamprecht, Sergio A., and Martin Lipkin. "Chemoprevention of colon cancer by calcium, vitamin D and folate: molecular mechanisms." *Nature Reviews Cancer* 3, no. 8 (2003): 601-614.

6. Treating Colorectal Cancer with Turmeric, Turmeric.com, http://www.turmeric.com/colorectal-cancer-treatment/treating-colorectal-cancer-with-turmeric

PART E
Avoid the Foods that Promote Cancer

Chapter 20: Sugar

1. Kroemer, Guido, and Jacques Pouyssegur. "Tumor cell metabolism: cancer's Achilles' heel." *Cancer cell* 13, no. 6 (2008): 472-482.

2. Jee, Sun Ha, Heechoul Ohrr, Jae Woong Sull, Ji Eun Yun, Min Ji, and Jonathan M. Samet. "Fasting serum glucose level and cancer risk in Korean men and women." *Jama* 293, no. 2 (2005): 194-202.

3. Cancer News, Articles, & Information, http://healthhubs.net/cancer/high-blood-sugar-levels-and-the-risk-of-cancer/

4. Johnson, J. A., B. Carstensen, D. Witte, S. L. Bowker, L. Lipscombe, A. G. Renehan, and Diabetes and Cancer Research Consortium. "Diabetes and cancer (1): evaluating the temporal relationship between type 2 diabetes and cancer incidence." *Diabetologia* 55, no. 6 (2012): 1607-1618.

5. Onodera, Yasuhito, Jin-Min Nam, and Mina J. Bissell. "Increased sugar uptake promotes oncogenesis via EPAC/RAP1

and O-GlcNAc pathways."*The Journal of clinical investigation* 124, no. 1 (2014): 367-384.

6. Erickson, Kirsten, Ruth E. Patterson, Shirley W. Flatt, Loki Natarajan, Barbara A. Parker, Dennis D. Heath, Gail A. Laughlin, Nazmus Saquib, Cheryl L. Rock, and John P. Pierce. "Clinically defined type 2 diabetes mellitus and prognosis in early-stage breast cancer." *Journal of Clinical Oncology* 29, no. 1 (2011): 54-60.

7. Hormones, The Endogenous, and Breast Cancer Collaborative Group. "Insulin-like growth factor 1 (IGF1), IGF binding protein 3 (IGFBP3), and breast cancer risk: pooled individual data analysis of 17 prospective studies."*The lancet oncology* 11, no. 6 (2010): 530-542.

8. Grothey, A., W. Voigt, C. Schöber, T. Müller, W. Dempke, and H. J. Schmoll. "The role of insulin-like growth factor I and its receptor in cell growth, transformation, apoptosis, and chemoresistance in solid tumors." *Journal of cancer research and clinical oncology* 125, no. 3-4 (1999): 166-173.

9. Leung, Cindy W., Barbara A. Laraia, Belinda L. Needham, David H. Rehkopf, Nancy E. Adler, Jue Lin, Elizabeth H. Blackburn, and Elissa S. Epel. "Soda and cell aging: associations between sugar-sweetened beverage consumption and leukocyte telomere length in healthy adults from the National Health and Nutrition Examination Surveys." *American journal of public health* 104, no. 12 (2014): 2425-2431.

10. Hu, J., C. La Vecchia, L. S. Augustin, E. Negri, M. De Groh, H. Morrison, L. Mery, and Canadian Cancer Registries Epidemiology Research Group. "Glycemic index, glycemic load and cancer risk." *Annals of oncology* (2012): mds235.

11. Galeone, Carlotta, Claudio Pelucchi, and Carlo La Vecchia. "Added sugar, glycemic index and load in colon cancer risk." *Current Opinion in Clinical Nutrition & Metabolic Care* 15, no. 4 (2012): 368-373.

12. Michaud, Dominique S., Simin Liu, Edward Giovannucci, Walter C. Willett, Graham A. Colditz, and Charles S. Fuchs. "Dietary sugar, glycemic load, and pancreatic cancer risk in a prospective study." *Journal of the National Cancer Institute* 94, no. 17 (2002): 1293-1300.

13. Belle, Fabiën N., Ellen Kampman, Anne McTiernan, Leslie Bernstein, Kathy Baumgartner, Richard Baumgartner, Anita Ambs, Rachel Ballard-Barbash, and Marian L. Neuhouser. "Dietary fiber, carbohydrates, glycemic index, and glycemic load in relation to breast cancer prognosis in the HEAL cohort."*Cancer Epidemiology Biomarkers & Prevention* 20, no. 5 (2011): 890-899.

14. Venkateswaran, Vasundara, Ahmed Q. Haddad, Neil E. Fleshner, Rong Fan, Linda M. Sugar, Rob Nam, Laurence H. Klotz, and Michael Pollak. "Association of diet-induced hyperinsulinemia with accelerated growth of prostate cancer (LNCaP) xenografts." *Journal of the National Cancer Institute*99, no. 23 (2007): 1793-1800.

15. Optimal Diets for Cancer Patients: 8 years of cancer survivor's best choices, Huber Colleen, NatureWorksBest Cancer Clinic, https://natureworksbest.com/wp-content/uploads/2015/12/Optimal-Diets-for-Cancer-Patients.pdf

16. Currie, Craig John, Christopher David Poole, and E. A. M. Gale. "The influence of glucose-lowering therapies on cancer risk in type 2 diabetes."*Diabetologia* 52, no. 9 (2009): 1766-1777.

17. Libby, Gillian, Louise A. Donnelly, Peter T. Donnan, Dario R. Alessi, Andrew D. Morris, and Josie MM Evans. "New Users of Metformin Are at Low Risk of Incident Cancer A cohort study among people with type 2 diabetes." *Diabetes care* 32, no. 9 (2009): 1620-1625.

Chapter 21: Caution with Eating Meat

1. World Cancer Research Fund / American Institute for Cancer Research (AICR). Food, nutrition, physical activity, and the prevention of cancer: a global perspective. Washington, DC: AICR; 2007

2. Derry, Molly Marie, Komal Raina, and Rajesh Agarwal. "Identifying molecular targets of lifestyle modifications in colon cancer prevention." *Frontiers in oncology* 3 (2013): 119.

3. Wei, Esther K., Graham A. Colditz, Edward L. Giovannucci, Charles S. Fuchs, and Bernard A. Rosner. "Cumulative risk of colon cancer up to age 70 years by risk factor status using data from the Nurses' Health Study."*American journal of epidemiology* 170, no. 7 (2009): 863-872.

4. Cross, Amanda J., Michael F. Leitzmann, Mitchell H. Gail, Albert R. Hollenbeck, Arthur Schatzkin, and Rashmi Sinha. "A prospective study of red and processed meat intake in relation to cancer risk." *PLoS Med* 4, no. 12 (2007): e325.

5. Rohrmann, Sabine, Kim Overvad, H. Bas Bueno-de-Mesquita, Marianne U. Jakobsen, Rikke Egeberg, Anne Tjønneland, Laura Nailler et al. "Meat consumption and mortality-results from the European Prospective Investigation into Cancer and Nutrition." *BMC medicine* 11, no. 1 (2013): 1.

6. Working, IARC Monograph. "Carcinogenicity of consumption of red and processed meat." (2015).

7. Zheng, Wei, and Sang-Ah Lee. "Well-done meat intake, heterocyclic amine exposure, and cancer risk." *Nutrition and cancer* 61, no. 4 (2009): 437-446.

8. Hebeisen, Dorothea F., F. Hoeflin, H. P. Reusch, E. Junker, and B. H. Lauterburg. "Increased concentrations of omega-3 fatty acids in milk and platelet rich plasma of grass-fed cows." *International journal for vitamin and nutrition research. Internationale Zeitschrift fur Vitamin-und Ernahrungsforschung. Journal international de vitaminologie et de nutrition*63, no. 3 (1992): 229-233.

9. Boada, Luis D., Marta Sangil, Eva E. Álvarez-León, Guayarmina Hernández-Rodríguez, Luis Alberto Henríquez-Hernández, María Camacho, Manuel Zumbado, Lluis Serra-Majem, and Octavio P. Luzardo. "Consumption of foods of animal origin as determinant of contamination by organochlorine pesticides and polychlorobiphenyls: results from a population-based study in Spain." *Chemosphere* 114 (2014): 121-128.

10. Kushi, Lawrence H., Tim Byers, Colleen Doyle, Elisa V. Bandera, Marji McCullough, Ted Gansler, Kimberly S. Andrews, and Michael J. Thun. "American Cancer Society Guidelines on Nutrition and Physical Activity for cancer prevention: reducing the risk of cancer with healthy food choices and physical activity." *CA: a cancer journal for clinicians* 56, no. 5 (2006): 254-281.

11. Daniel, Carrie R., Amanda J. Cross, Barry I. Graubard, Albert R. Hollenbeck, Yikyung Park, and Rashmi Sinha. "Prospective investigation of poultry and fish intake in relation to cancer risk." *Cancer Prevention Research* 4, no. 11 (2011): 1903-1911.

12. Khan, Mohammad Rizwan, Rosa Busquets, Javier Saurina, Santiago Hernández, and Lluís Puignou. "Identification of seafood as an important dietary source of heterocyclic amines by chemometry and chromatography–mass spectrometry." *Chemical research in toxicology* 26, no. 6 (2013): 1014-1022.

13. Joshi, Amit D., Esther M. John, Jocelyn Koo, Sue A. Ingles, and Mariana C. Stern. "Fish intake, cooking practices, and risk of prostate cancer: results from a multi-ethnic case–control study." *Cancer Causes & Control* 23, no. 3 (2012): 405-420.

14. Torfadottir, Johanna E., Unnur A. Valdimarsdottir, Lorelei A. Mucci, Julie L. Kasperzyk, Katja Fall, Laufey Tryggvadottir, Thor Aspelund et al. "Consumption of fish products across the lifespan and prostate cancer risk." *PloS one* 8, no. 4 (2013): e59799.

15. Key, Timothy J., Paul N. Appleby, Francesca L. Crowe, Kathryn E. Bradbury, Julie A. Schmidt, and Ruth C. Travis. "Cancer in British vegetarians: updated analyses of 4998 incident cancers in a cohort of 32,491 meat eaters, 8612 fish eaters, 18,298 vegetarians, and 2246 vegans." *The American journal of clinical nutrition* 100, no. Supplement 1 (2014): 378S-385S.

16. Tantamango-Bartley, Yessenia, Karen Jaceldo-Siegl, Jing Fan, and Gary Fraser. "Vegetarian diets and the incidence of cancer in a low-risk population." *Cancer Epidemiology Biomarkers & Prevention* 22, no. 2 (2013): 286-294.

17. Orlich, Michael J., Pramil N. Singh, Joan Sabaté, Jing Fan, Lars Sveen, Hannelore Bennett, Synnove F. Knutsen et al. "Vegetarian dietary patterns and the risk of colorectal cancers." *JAMA internal medicine* 175, no. 5 (2015): 767-776.

Chapter 22: Acrylamide

1. The heatox project, www.heatox.org, HEATOX, Heat generated food toxicants: identification, characterization and risk minimization, http://www.elika.eus/datos/articulos/Archivo266/Heatox_InforFINAL07.pdf

2. HEATOX project completed – brings new pieces to the Acrylamide Puzzle, Press Release November 2007, http://ec.europa.eu/research/index.cfm?pg=newsalert&year=2007&na=na-261107

Chapter 23: Reduce Cancer Risk by Reducing Dietary Salt

1. Kiwon Kim, Nephrology Clinic, National Cancer Center, slideshow accessed at: http://www.slideshare.net/KiwonKim/salt-and-cancer-risk

2. Peleteiro, B., C. Lopes, C. Figueiredo, and N. Lunet. "Salt intake and gastric cancer risk according to Helicobacter pylori

infection, smoking, tumour site and histological type." *British journal of cancer* 104, no. 1 (2011): 198-207.

3. Ge, Sheng, Xiaohui Feng, Li Shen, Zhanying Wei, Qiankun Zhu, and Juan Sun. "Association between habitual dietary salt intake and risk of gastric cancer: a systematic review of observational studies." *Gastroenterology research and practice* 2012 (2012).

Chapter 24: Foods that Cause Inflammation and Their Relationship with Cancer

1. Riccio, Paolo, and Rocco Rossano. "Nutrition facts in multiple sclerosis." *ASN neuro* 7, no. 1 (2015): 1759091414568185.

2. Heidland, August, André Klassen, Przemyslaw Rutkowski, and Udo Bahner. "The contribution of Rudolf Virchow to the concept of inflammation: what is still of importance?." *Journal of nephrology* 19, no. 3 (2006): S102.

3. Eiró, Noemí, and Francisco J. Vizoso. "Inflammation and cancer." *World J Gastrointest Surg* 4, no. 3 (2012): 62-72

4. Grivennikov, Sergei I., Florian R. Greten, and Michael Karin. "Immunity, inflammation, and cancer." *Cell* 140, no. 6 (2010): 883-899.

5. Pierce, Brandon L., Rachel Ballard-Barbash, Leslie Bernstein, Richard N. Baumgartner, Marian L. Neuhouser, Mark H. Wener, Kathy B. Baumgartner et al. "Elevated biomarkers of inflammation are associated with reduced survival among breast cancer patients." *Journal of Clinical Oncology* 27, no. 21 (2009): 3437-3444.

6. Grivennikov, Sergei I., Florian R. Greten, and Michael Karin. "Immunity, inflammation, and cancer." *Cell* 140, no. 6 (2010): 883-899.

7. Grivennikov, Sergei I., Florian R. Greten, and Michael Karin. "Immunity, inflammation, and cancer." *Cell* 140, no. 6 (2010): 883-899.

8. Riccio, Paolo, and Rocco Rossano. "Nutrition facts in multiple sclerosis." *ASN neuro* 7, no. 1 (2015): 1759091414568185.
9. Pro-Inflammatory Diet Linked to Colorectal Cancer, Poor Metabolic Health. American Institute for Cancer research, http://www.aicr.org/press/press-releases/2014/pro-inflammatory-diet-linked-to-colorectal-cancer-poor-metabolic-health.html
10. Shivappa, Nitin, Anna E. Prizment, Cindy K. Blair, David R. Jacobs, Susan E. Steck, and James R. Hébert. "Dietary inflammatory index and risk of colorectal cancer in the Iowa Women's Health Study." *Cancer Epidemiology Biomarkers & Prevention* 23, no. 11 (2014): 2383-2392.
11. Susan E. Steck, Fred K. Tabung, Michael D. Wirth, Academy of Nutrition and Dietetics, The Digest, "The Dietary Inflammatory Index: A new tool for Assessing Diet Quality Based on Inflammatory Potential", Vol. 49, Number 3 (2014)

Chapter 25: Unhealthy Fats: Excess Omega-6

1. Optimize omega-6 to omega-3 ratio, Authority Nutrition, http://authoritynutrition.com/optimize-omega-6-omega-3-ratio/
2. Simopoulos, A. P. "Evolutionary aspects of diet, the omega-6/omega-3 ratio and genetic variation: nutritional implications for chronic diseases."*Biomedicine & pharmacotherapy* 60, no. 9 (2006): 502-507.
3. Anti-cancer Nutrition: Dietary Fats 101, Integrative Oncology Essentials, http://www.integrativeoncology-essentials.com/2012/10/anti-cancer-nutrition-dietary-fats-101/
4. Kiage, James N., Peter D. Merrill, Cody J. Robinson, Yue Cao, Talha A. Malik, Barrett C. Hundley, Ping Lao et al. "Intake of trans fat and all-cause mortality in the Reasons for Geographical and Racial Differences in Stroke (REGARDS) cohort." *The American journal of clinical nutrition* 97, no. 5 (2013): 1121-1128.

5. Chajès, Véronique, Anne CM Thiébaut, Maxime Rotival, Estelle Gauthier, Virginie Maillard, Marie-Christine Boutron-Ruault, Virginie Joulin, Gilbert M. Lenoir, and Françoise Clavel-Chapelon. "Association between serum trans-monounsaturated fatty acids and breast cancer risk in the E3N-EPIC Study."*American journal of epidemiology* 167, no. 11 (2008): 1312-1320.
6. Anti-cancer Nutrition: Dietary Fats 101, Integrative Oncology Essentials, http://www.integrativeoncology-essentials.com/2012/10/anti-cancer-nutrition-dietary-fats-101/

Chapter 26: Food Additives Causing Inflammation

1. Carrageenan: How a "natural" food additive is making us sick. A report by The Cornucopia Institute, March 2013
2. Tobacman, Joanne K. "Review of harmful gastrointestinal effects of carrageenan in animal experiments." *Environmental health perspectives* 109, no. 10 (2001): 983.
3. Carrageenan: How a "natural" food additive is making us sick. A report by The Cornucopia Institute, March 2013
4. http://www.cornucopia.org/2013/12/carrageenan-risks-reality/

Chapter 27: Exposure to Environmental and Dietary Carcinogens

1. National Cancer Institute, President's Cancer Panel, Reducing Environmental Cancer Risk, What We Can Do Now, (2010), http://deainfo.nci.nih.gov/advisory/pcp/annualReports/pcp08-09rpt/PCP_Report_08-09_508.pdf
2. Cancer-causing substances in the environment, National Cancer Institute, http://www.cancer.gov/about-cancer/causes-prevention/risk/substances
3. http://articles.mercola.com/sites/articles/archive/2015/12/08/toxic-chemical-health-risks.aspx

4. Goodson, William H., Leroy Lowe, David O. Carpenter, Michael Gilbertson, Abdul Manaf Ali, Adela Lopez de Cerain Salsamendi, Ahmed Lasfar et al. "Assessing the carcinogenic potential of low-dose exposures to chemical mixtures in the environment: the challenge ahead." *Carcinogenesis* 36, no. Suppl 1 (2015): S254-S296.

5. Food and Drug Administration. Bad Bug Book, Foodborne Pathogenic Microorganisms and Natural Toxins, Second Edition. Laurel, MD (2012)

6. International Agency for Research on Cancer. Aflatoxins, IARC Monographs on the Evaluation of Carcinogenic Risks to Humans, Volume 100F. Lyon, France: World Health Organization (2012)

7. Barrett, Julia R. "Liver cancer and aflatoxin: New information from the Kenyan outbreak." *Environmental health perspectives* 113, no. 12 (2005): A837.

8. Arsenic in Rice: Should you be concerned? Authority Nutrition, http://authority nutrition.com/arsenic-in-rice/

9. Arsenic, WHO, (2016), http://www.who.int/mediacentre/factsheets/fs372/en/

10. Arsenic, National Cancer Institute, http://www.cancer.gov/about-cancer/causes-prevention /risk/substances/arsenic

11. Arsenic, WHO, (2016), http://www.who.int/mediacentre/factsheets/fs372/en/

12. Arsenic, National Cancer Institute, http://www.cancer.gov/about-cancer/causes-prevention /risk/substances/arsenic

13. Simple cooking methods flush arsenic out of rice, Nature, (2015), http://www.nature.com/news/simple-cooking-methods-flush-arsenic-out-of-rice-1.18034

14. What is BPA, and what are the concerns about BPA?, Mayo Clinic, http://www.mayoclinic.org/healthy-lifestyle/nutrition- and-healthy-eating/expert-answers/bpa/faq-20058331

15. Lozada, Kristen Weber, and Ruth A. Keri. "Bisphenol A increases mammary cancer risk in two distinct mouse models of breast cancer." *Biology of reproduction* 85, no. 3 (2011): 490-497.

16. Lozada, Kristen Weber, and Ruth A. Keri. "Bisphenol A increases mammary cancer risk in two distinct mouse models of breast cancer." *Biology of reproduction* 85, no. 3 (2011): 490-497.

17. Prins, Gail S. "Endocrine disruptors and prostate cancer risk." *Endocrine-Related Cancer* 15, no. 3 (2008): 649-656.

18. BPA increases risk of cancer in human prostate tissue, UIC news, (2014), https://news.uic.edu/bpa-increases-risk-of-cancer-in-human-prostate-tissue

19. New study confirms BOA in receipts, EWG (2010), http://www.ewg.org/research/new-study-confirms-bpa-receipts

20. Phthalates, Breast Cancer Fund, breastcancerfund.org/clear-science/biology-of-breast-cancer/endocrine-disrupting-compounds

21. Phthalates, Canadian Cancer Society, http://www.cancer.ca/en/prevention-and-screening/be-aware/harmful-substances-and-environmental-risks/phthalates/

22. Non-stick cookware, Canadian Cancer Society, http://www.cancer.ca/en/prevention-and-screening/be-aware/harmful-substances-and-environmental-risks/non-stick-cookware

23. Steenland, Kyle, Tony Fletcher, and David A. Savitz. "Epidemiologic evidence on the health effects of perfluorooctanoic acid (PFOA)." *Environmental health perspectives* (2010): 1100-1108.

24. Teflon-and-perfluorooctanoic-acid—pfoa, American Cancer Society, http://www.cancer.org/cancer/cancercauses/othercarcinogens/athome/teflon-and-perfluorooctanoic-acid--pfoa

25. C8 Science Panel, http://www.c8sciencepanel.org/index.html

26. Probable link evaluation of cancer, Science Panel (2012c), C8 Probable Link Reports. http://www.c8sciencepanel.org/pdfs/ Probable_Link_C8_Cancer_16April2012_v2.pdf

27. Dioxins, Breast Cancer Fund, http://www.breastcancerfund. org/clear-science/radiation-chemicals-and-breast-cancer/dioxins.html

28. IARC Monographs on the evaluation of carcinogenic risks to humans, http://monographs.iarc.fr/ENG/Monographs/vol69/

29. Learn about Dioxin, US Environmental Protection Agency, http://www2.epa.gov /dioxin/learn-about-dioxin

30. Dioxins and dioxin-like compounds, Wikipedia, https://en.wikipedia.org/wiki/ Dioxins_and_dioxin-like_compounds

31. Stockholm convention on Persistent Organic Pollutants, https:// en.wikipedia.org/wiki/Stockholm_Convention_on_Persistent_Organic_Pollutants

32. Nøstbakken, Ole Jakob, Helge T. Hove, Arne Duinker, Anne-Katrine Lundebye, Marc HG Berntssen, Rita Hannisdal, Bjørn Tore Lunestad et al. "Contaminant levels in Norwegian farmed Atlantic salmon (Salmo salar) in the 13-year period from 1999 to 2011." *Environment international* 74 (2015): 274-280.

33. Dioxin, Environmental Protection Agency, http://www3.epa. gov/airtoxics/hlthef /dioxin.html

34. Foran, Jeffery A., David O. Carpenter, M. Coreen Hamilton, Barbara A. Knuth, and Steven J. Schwager. "Risk-based consumption advice for farmed Atlantic and wild Pacific salmon contaminated with dioxins and dioxin-like compounds." *Environmental health perspectives* (2005): 552-556.

35. Sweden sells toxic Baltic salmon to EU, The Local, http://www. thelocal.se/20130508

36. /47782

37. Fishupdate, Salmon scandal causes stir in Sweden – Fishupdate.com, http://www.fishupdate.com/

38. salmon-schttp://www.bbc.com/news/world-europe-22446780an-dal-causes-stir-in-sweden-fishupdate-com/ on 10 August 2016

39. BBC News, Swedish salmon sales 'breached EU ban' over dioxins, 8 May 2013, http://www.bbc.com/news/world-europe-22446780

40. Nøstbakken, Ole Jakob, Helge T. Hove, Arne Duinker, Anne-Katrine Lundebye, Marc HG Berntssen, Rita Hannisdal, Bjørn Tore Lunestad et al. "Contaminant levels in Norwegian farmed Atlantic salmon (Salmo salar) in the 13-year period from 1999 to 2011." *Environment international* 74 (2015): 274-280.

41. http://alexandramorton.typepad.com/alexandra_morton/2013/12/dear-whole-foods-toxins-in-your-farmed-salmon.html

42. Pesticides, Canadian Cancer Society, http://www.cancer.ca/en/prevention-and-screening/be-aware/harmful-substances-and-environmental-risks/pesticides

43. Pesticides, Canadian Cancer Society, http://www.cancer.ca/en/prevention-and-screening/be-aware/harmful-substances-and-environmental-risks/pesticides

44. EWG's 2016 Shopper's Guide to Pesticides in Produce, http://www.ewg.org/foodnews /summary.php

45. Chlorinated water, Canadian Cancer Society, http://www.cancer.ca/en/prevention-and-screening/be-aware/harmful-substances-and-environmental-risks/chlorinated-water

46. Pelucchi, Claudio, Irene Tramacere, Paolo Boffetta, Eva Negri, and Carlo La Vecchia. "Alcohol consumption and cancer risk." *Nutrition and cancer* 63, no. 7 (2011): 983-990.

47. 9 in 10 don't link alcohol and cancer, Cancer Research UK, http://www.cancerresearchuk.org/about-us/cancer-news/press-release/2016-04-01-9-in-10-dont-link-alcohol-and-cancer

48. Alcohol use and cancer, American Cancer Society, http://www.cancer.org/cancer/cancercauses/dietandphysicalactivity/alcohol-use-and-cancer

49. Dr David Servan-Schreiber, Anti-Cancer : A new Way of life, Penguin Books, ISBN: 978-0-718-15684-8

PART F:
Toxin Removal and Physical Activity

Chapter 28: Enhance Your Ability to Remove Toxins

1. Metabolic Detoxification, Life Extension, http://www.lifeextension.com/protocols/ metabolic-health/metabolic-detoxification/Page-01

2. Life Extension Disease Prevemtion and Treatment, 5th Edition, 2013, ISBN 978-0-9658777-8-7

3. Rayman, Margaret P. "Selenium in cancer prevention: a review of the evidence and mechanism of action." *Proceedings of the Nutrition Society* 64, no. 04 (2005): 527-542.

4. Ramasamy, Kumaraguruparan, and Rajesh Agarwal. "Multi-targeted therapy of cancer by silymarin." *Cancer letters* 269, no. 2 (2008): 352-362.

5. Ramasamy, Kumaraguruparan, and Rajesh Agarwal. "Multi-targeted therapy of cancer by silymarin." *Cancer letters* 269, no. 2 (2008): 352-362.

6. Klein, A. V., and H. Kiat. "Detox diets for toxin elimination and weight management: a critical review of the evidence." *Journal of Human Nutrition and Dietetics* 28, no. 6 (2015): 675-686.

7. Sears, Margaret E. "Chelation: harnessing and enhancing heavy metal detoxification—a review." *The Scientific World Journal* 2013 (2013).

8. Aga, Miho, Kanso Iwaki, Yasuto Ueda, Shimpei Ushio, Naoya Masaki, Shigeharu Fukuda, Tetsuo Kimoto, Masao Ikeda, and Masashi Kurimoto. "Preventive effect of Coriandrum sativum (Chinese parsley) on localized lead deposition in ICR mice." *Journal of ethnopharmacology* 77, no. 2 (2001): 203-208.

9. Sharma, Veena, Leena Kansal, and Arti Sharma. "Prophylactic efficacy of Coriandrum sativum (Coriander) on testis of lead-exposed mice." *Biological trace element research* 136, no. 3 (2010): 337-354.

10. Kim, Jung Hee, Hye Bog Na, and Mi Joung Kim. "Effects of the lemon detox program on body fat reduction and detoxification in Korean overweight women (LB354)." *The FASEB Journal* 28, no. 1 Supplement (2014): LB354.

11. Kim, Jung Hee, Hye Bog Na, and Mi Joung Kim. "Effects of the lemon detox program on body fat reduction and detoxification in Korean overweight women (LB354)." *The FASEB Journal* 28, no. 1 Supplement (2014): LB354.

12. Superfoods for Optimum Health: Chlorella and Spirulina, Mike Adams, Truth Publishing International, http://www.naturalpharmainternational.com/1/upload/1803065_

13. superfoods_for_optimum_health_chlorella_spirulina_ mike_adams_truth_publishing.pdf

14. Metabolic Detoxification, Life Extension, http://www.lifeextension.com/protocols/metabolic-health/metabolic-detoxification/ Page-01

Chapter 29: Physical Activity: A Powerful Weapon against Cancer

1. Does Exercise Help Cancer Survivors? American Institute for Cancer Research Blog, http://blog.aicr.org/2014/10/30/ does-exercise-help-cancer-patients-and-survivors/

2. Physical Activity and Cancer Risk, Cancer.Net, http://www.cancer.net/navigating-cancer-care/prevention-and-healthy-living/physical-activity-and-cancer-risk

3. American Cancer Society guidelines on nutrition and physical activity for cancer prevention, http://www.cancer.org/acs/ groups/cid/documents/webcontent/002577-pdf.pdf

4. Friedenreich, Christine M., Qinggang Wang, Heather K. Neilson, Karen A. Kopciuk, S. Elizabeth McGregor, and Kerry S. Courneya. "Physical activity and survival after prostate cancer." *European urology* (2016).

5. Beasley, Jeannette M., Marilyn L. Kwan, Wendy Y. Chen, Erin K. Weltzien, Candyce H. Kroenke, Wei Lu, Sarah J. Nechuta et al. "Meeting the physical activity guidelines and survival after breast cancer: findings from the after breast cancer pooling project." *Breast cancer research and treatment* 131, no. 2 (2012): 637-643.

6. American Cancer Society guidelines on nutrition and physical activity for cancer prevention, http://www.cancer.org/acs/groups/cid/documents/webcontent/002577-pdf.pdf

7. Physical Activity Guidelines Advisory Committee. "Physical activity guidelines advisory committee report, 2008." *Washington, DC: US Department of Health and Human Services* 2008 (2008): A1-H14.

8. Blood glucose control and exercise, American Diabetes Association, http://www.diabetes. org/food-and-fitness/fitness/get-started-safely/blood-glucose-control-and-exercise.html

9. Stocks, T., Rapp, K., Bjørge, T., Manjer, J., Ulmer, H., Selmer, R., Lukanova, A., Johansen, D., Concin, H., Tretli, S. and Hallmans, G., 2009. Blood glucose and risk of incident and fatal cancer in the metabolic syndrome and cancer project (me-can): analysis of six prospective cohorts. *PLoS Med*, 6(12), p.e1000201.

10. Kruijsen-Jaarsma, Mirjam, Dóra Révész, Marc B. Bierings, Laurien M. Buffart, and Tim Takken. "Effects of exercise on immune function in patients with cancer: a systematic review." *Exerc Immunol Rev* 19 (2013): 120-143.